Acupuncture: The Limericks

Acupuncture: The Limericks

an introduction to acupuncture

Cornelia Davies BAc (UK), Cert Ac (Beijing)

Golden Barn Publishing
UK

First published 2009
by Golden Barn Publishing , UK
www.acupuncturekingsbridge.co.uk

Text design by Roger Lane

Cover design by Brian Weldon and Chandler Design

Printed in Great Britain by the MPG Books Group, Bodmin and King's Lynn, on paper produced using a chlorine-free process

Disclaimer

My disclaimer says this, in the main,
"Please desist from, resist and refrain...
Don't put pins in at home
When you've finished this tome—
You might painfully puncture a vein."

Which means: The contents of this book are for information only. The author recommends that you consult qualified practitioners when considering treatment. Do not attempt to self-treat or alter your medication without consulting a doctor. The author and publisher cannot accept responsibility for illness or injury arising from a failure to follow these guidelines.

Dedication

To all my acupuncture teachers and patients, past, present and future, for inspiring me in the practice of this wonderful system of medicine.

Acknowledgements

With heartfelt thanks to Jane Robinson for encouraging me to write this book, and for her technical proofreading.

My thanks are also due to to Celia Warren, Diane Whitaker and Colm O'Rourke for proofreading, to Roger Lane for help with formatting, and to numerous friends and colleagues for their enthusiasm.

My appreciation goes to the friends who have allowed me photograph them. Unless credited, photos are taken by the author. Thanks for permission to use additional photos by Jane Body and Carl Hahn.

Cover image from a painting by Xiao Bai Li.
Author cover photo by Celia Warren.

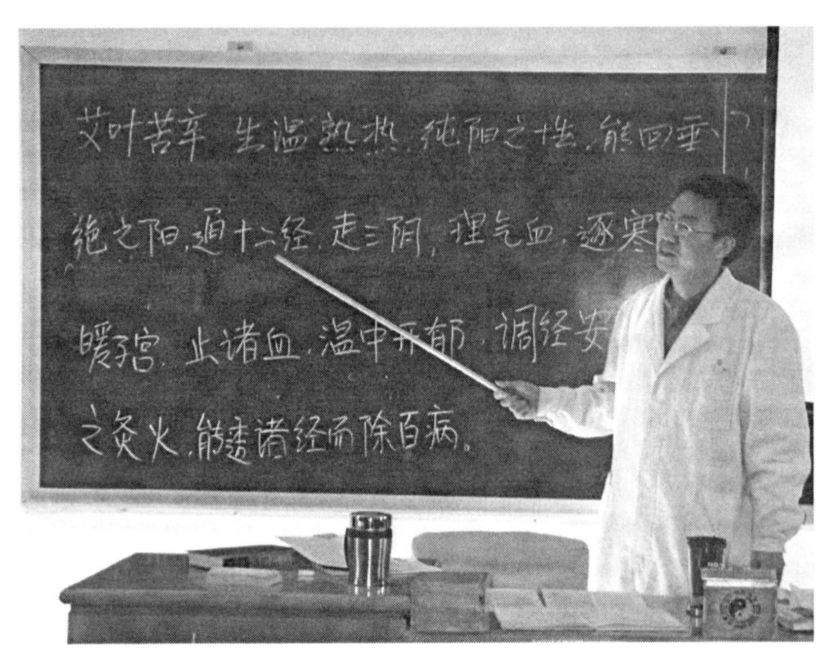

Here's one of my wonderful teachers in China showing the class a traditional verse used by Chinese students to memorize the uses of moxa

Foreword

In China, the students of old
Studied meekly with teachers who'd scold,
So, immersed in some verse,
They would tersely rehearse
Till their knowledge became purest gold.

Traditionally, trainee acupuncture doctors in China used to learn poems, in order to memorize the principles of their subject, so it's not so mad to have a book of limericks about acupuncture in the modern day.

My intention is that you will enjoy reading these verses and that they will open up your awareness of this remarkable system of medicine, which is as relevant nowadays in the West as it has been in China for thousands of years.

So read freely this limerick verse—
You've no need to feel worried or curse,
As you don't have, for teachers,
Vindictive old creatures…
Relax, guys, your lives could be worse!

Author's Note

When a biological term is used in its Chinese medical context, each word is written with upper case beginning letter(s) and *italicised*. When it is used in the Western sense, upper case and italics are not used.

Examples:

Heart meridian (as in Chinese medicine)
heart (referring to the organ)
Gall Bladder (the function in Chinese medicine)
gall bladder (the organ in Western medicine)

Blood (the substance, in Chinese medicine)
blood (as in Western medicine)

Other specialist words are italicised.

Chinese and Greek terms are ***italicised and in boldface***

Examples:

Qi *(life force)*
Shen Men *(Spirit Door)*
alpha *waves*

Contents

Acupuncture is Part of Chinese Medicine

Chinese medicine—now where do I start?
Acupuncture and herbs play a part,
As do ***tui na*** and ***moxa***;
And *cupping* unlocks a
New level of health—what an art!

There are many different skills involved in the practice of Chinese medicine.

Probably the best-known component is acupuncture, in which incredibly fine needles are used to remove blockages to health. A complete differential diagnosis is made prior to adjusting the flow of ***Qi*** (pronounced *chee*, and meaning *energy* or *life force*) in the acupuncture *meridians* (channels of energy). Chinese herbal medicine also uses this elegant and far-reaching form of diagnosis. ***Tui na*** is Chinese massage.

Moxibustion (***moxa***) is a warming technique, which involves burning medicinal herbs, safely, near to the patient to guide warmth into the body, and which also explains the strange burning smell you might encounter in an acupuncture clinic.

Cupping is a fire treatment, using glass *cups* to create a vacuum to relax and warm muscles. It moves stagnation within the body and stimulates the immune system. This is very helpful for people with back, shoulder, hip and knee problems and is also useful when you are going down with a cold.

A young person had reason for sneezing
With cold (she was practically freezing).
Some *cups* on her back
Helped repel the attack:
Now her wheezing is easing… how pleasing.

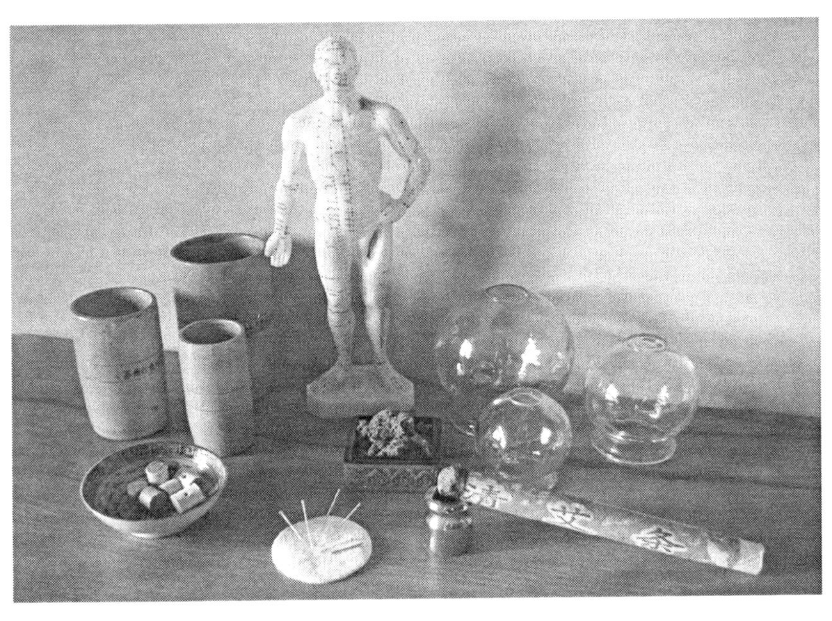

A selection of equipment: traditional bamboo cupping jars, a model showing the acupuncture meridians, glass cupping jars, mini moxa rolls, acupuncture needles, loose moxa in a container & a moxa roll

The Needles

The needles of steel are hair-thin,
Bringing ease when they're carefully in.
Every needle is new
And disposable—true:
After treatment it's chucked in a bin.

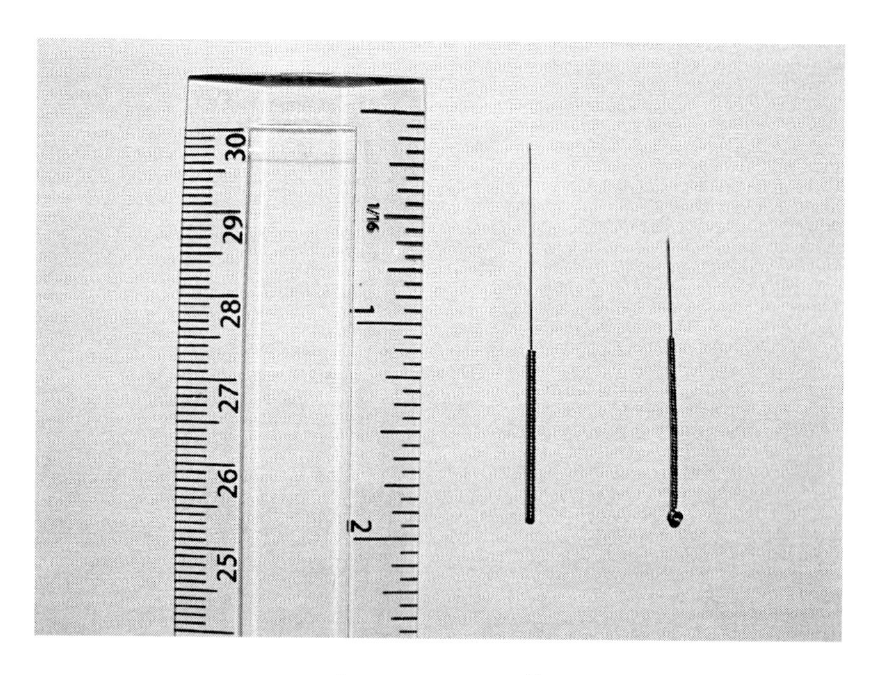

Acupuncture needles

Yes, all acupuncture needles used in the Western world are disposable, which also eliminates the risk of cross infection. The 'sharps' disposal bins are collected by licensed companies for safe disposal.

Compared to injection, or even sewing needles, acupuncture needles are tiny. They are made of stainless steel, and they really are nearly as thin as hairs. They are flexible and do not break.

If you've joint pain or migraine, then pitch up
At your therapist's place, and then hitch up
Your sleeve for relief,
But forget the belief
That the needles will feel like a stitch-up.

To avoid unnecessary discomfort to the patient, acupuncturists are taught to insert the needles extremely quickly through the sensitive skin layer. Once under the skin, in order for the treatment to be effective, each needle must make contact with the acupuncture point. This is a tiny, precisely defined area just below the surface. It connects with the overall web of ***Qi*** (*chee: energy* or *life force*), which runs throughout the body. This allows blocked energy to be cleared and deficiency or excess in the body to be balanced.

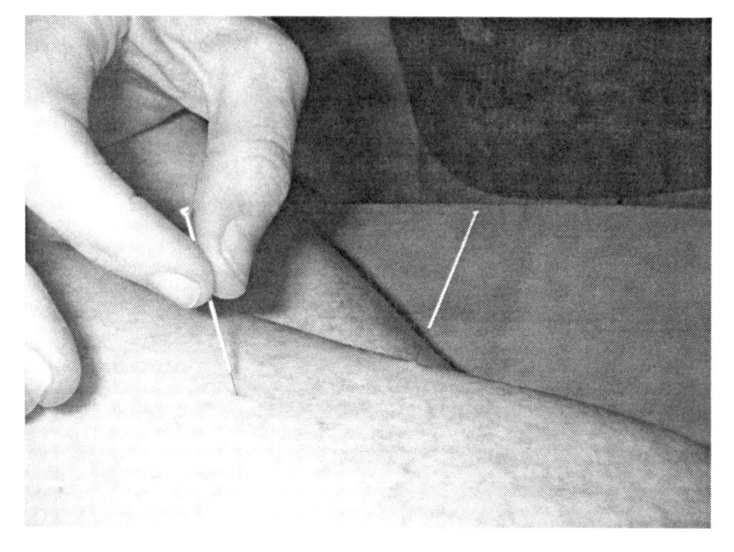

Photo Carl Hahn

When the needle touches the *acu point*, the patient is usually aware of a special sensation. This is different from what is felt with an injection or even a pinprick. It can be described as being rather like an *electrical* sensation. This feeling does not usually last long, but it's great that it happens, as it gives a very clear idea of what is occurring at the energy, or ***Qi*** *(chee)*, level.

"Dr Pins, tell me how will it be,
When you place those small needles in me?"
"You may sense some electric—
Though that could sound eccentric,
It describes the connection with ***Qi***."

Generally, the needles will be left in place for ten to thirty minutes, though sometimes they are removed immediately. When young children and babies are treated, the needles are always removed straight away.

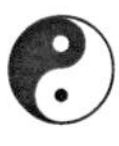

The Ballad of the Bian Stone Needle

Caveman Dayna's cool cousin, Shu Lin,
Who's from China, invented a pin.
It was **thin as a rock**—
That's a term that could shock,
For a needle that pierces the skin.

Acupuncture is what Shu Lin uses,
And ***Bian Stone***, the needle he chooses,
But to practise on Dayna,
He hears the refrain, a
Tad sad, as our caveman refuses.

"Sharp rocks are as good as you'll get,"
Says Shu Lin to our man, "So get set:
And I'll tell you for free,
It's five thousand BC:
Stainless steel will take centuries yet!"

Then as time moved along, tools got thinner,
Till needles of bone proved a winner.
When no pain was excused,
Gold and silver were used,
And now steel is routinely the pinner.

Yes, all this is true about the ***Bian Stone*** (*bee-an stone*) needle. These acupuncture artefacts have been found dating back to about 5,000 BC. Though they are very thin, as far as *stone* goes, I do sometimes wonder if they were used to massage acupuncture points, rather than actually pierce the skin, but it seems unlikely that we'll ever know.

Later, needles of bone, jade, silver and gold were used, and nowadays, I'm relieved to say, we use disposable stainless steel ones.

Shu Lin (*shoo lin*) and Caveman Dayna are two fictional New Stone Age characters… but maybe they're not so fictional, as you'll find out at the end of this book.

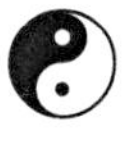

What Does the Patient Think?

At first I felt flustered and scared
As my arm, I reluctantly bared,
But Doc Pins is so kind,
That I'm fine—I don't mind:
I feel great and I'm glad that I dared.

It's true that quite a number of new patients feel nervous about their first treatment. Some of this is good old fear of the unknown… and, of course, some of it is fear of those needles. Well, the good news is that the needles are smaller than you might expect (they're certainly smaller than I imagined before my first treatment). The other piece of excellent news is that acupuncturists tend to be people who care about how other people feel, so they'll go out of their way to make you feel comfortable. They'll explain about the treatment and answer your questions, and will know that you might be anxious.

Something that may surprise you is that, once you get over any initial fears, you'll probably relax on the treatment couch (yes, with the needles in place!) After the first session, if you need some 'down' time during treatment, once the needles are in your practitioner may sit very quietly in the background, or may leave the room for a short while, if you feel comfortable with that. On returning after five or ten minutes, it's not uncommon to find a patient admitting that they have been snoozing.

If I'm tired beyond needing a rest,
Acupuncture's the answer – the best.
The treatment's good news:
I relax and then snooze,
And wake bouncy and fit—full of zest!

And feel?

I lie comfortably close to the brink
Of a dreamland and sleepily think,
"Is my visual sense true?
In my head I see blue
And it's morphing through purple to pink."

Some people describe seeing swirling colours in front of their closed eyes as they relax on the couch during a treatment. Not everyone sees colours, but many people do drop into a state of relaxation.

Acupuncture shares many experiential components with other forms of natural healing, and researchers have found a way to measure, scientifically, what happens to a patient during the healing process. They connect the person to an electroencephalograph (EEG), a machine that records brainwave patterns.

Being pinned to improve on your health, a
Remarkable thing creeps, with stealth: a
Profound sense of calm,
Which can soothe like a balm
As your brainwaves relax into ***alpha***.

Your brainwaves have different patterns depending on what psycho-physical state you're in. In your everyday, action-filled life, you operate using brainwaves called ***beta waves***. Being 'in' ***beta*** allows you to make decisions and act swiftly.

As you relax, say in a warm bath or sitting happily in the garden on a summer's evening, you slip into ***alpha waves.*** This allows your body-mind some much-needed 'down' time, and the chance to make running repairs. One of the reasons stress frequently leads to poor health is that when you go through a stressful time you tend to have less physical and/or emotional 'down' time .

Then there are ***theta waves***, which could be described as dream waves. When you are fortunate enough to slip into ***theta***, your body-mind can access an even deeper level of healing. When you are on the edge of sleep and experience fragments of semi-waking dream you are in ***theta*** brainwaves.

When your body relaxes to meet a,
Calm state, as your brainwaves leave ***beta***,
Allowing more healing,
Embracing a feeling,
Remarkably dreamy: that's ***theta***.

When you receive acupuncture, as the therapy is working, it's quite likely that at some time your brain will drop from *everyday* ***beta waves*** into *relaxing* ***alpha*** or even *dreamy* ***theta.*** Some people are conscious of this change in brainwaves and some are not so aware… and that's ok.

Don't worry if you don't feel things 'happening' during treatment. But if you're one of those people who sees colours or you feel that you become physically heavier and sink into the treatment couch, this is normal… don't panic, it's a good thing! The drop into ***alpha*** or ***theta*** waves allows for a more profound and lasting benefit at a cellular level, and this is great news for body, mind *and* spirit.

What's it feel like? I'll give you some facts:
You may comfortably sink and relax
While your mind isn't 'revvy',
Your limbs may feel heavy—
In brief, you'll feel lighter… untaxed.

Qi, Meridians and Points… Energy Talk

First there's Qi...

Acupuncturists talk of a force
Of great energy—well, where's its source?
They describe it as ***Qi***—
Tell me, what can that be?
Oh, invisible life force, of course!

Yes, we acupuncturists do have a habit of talking about ***Qi*** (pronounced *chee*) as though everyone else knows what we're on about! It's one of the foundations of our work, so you can't really blame us.

Qi can best be described as *life force*. It's that invisible substance that courses through our bodies to keep us alive. Eastern science has long had an explanation for this, and acupuncture theory has a clear outline of where and how ***Qi*** runs, at least to a level at which this knowledge can be useful in treatment.

There are two systems of transliterating Chinese into Western letters. The older system is known as *Wade-Giles*, in which the word for *life force* would be ***Chi*** (as in ***Tai Chi*** exercise). In modern-day China the system is called ***pinyin***, in which the same ***Chi*** becomes ***Qi.*** This tends to be the style used in Chinese medicine. In Japanese, while similar characters are used for writing, the pronunciation is a little different, so ***Chi*** becomes ***Ki*** *(kee).*

Chinese Qi can be written as Chi—
In Japan, though, they say it as Ki.
If the two are combined,
Like a rounded behind,
They are *Chee-Ky*— so diction is key.

...and meridians

Your *meridians* run true and free
Through your body, on paths we agree
Have been shown to exist
On a time-honoured list,
While transporting your life force: your ***Qi***.

Meridian pathways have been clearly mapped out for several centuries. There are fourteen main ones, which feed ***Qi*** energy to every part of the body. You could imagine these as being rather like invisible blood vessels, which, instead of carrying blood, carry *life force.*

The *Bladder* goes head down to toes;
Large Intestine ends close to the nose,
While the *Lung* is quite short—
Are these organs? As taught?
They're *meridians*: where the ***Qi*** flows.

Eleven of the fourteen main *meridians* have names which relate to the bodily organs they're connected with, but they cover a much more extensive area. For example, the *Bladder meridian* does have a branch that goes into the physical bladder, but it also stretches from your eye, over your head, right down your back and legs, and ends next to your little toe nail. This means that it's used in many cases of backache, cramp and a whole host of other conditions, as it has strong connections with all the organs. Other *meridians* are less extensive, in varying degrees, but they all have many important uses.

If you're fat, or just right, or quite thin,
You'll have *acu* points under your skin.
Every point has some links
To a web, which, methinks
Is like railway lines nestled within.

"So what exactly are these points and *meridians*?" is a usual question during treatment. We've already discovered that *meridians* are the channels that transport ***Qi*** (*life force*) around the body. When they get blocked or in some way, unbalanced, the slow, but sure, course of illness begins. The ancient Chinese identified acupuncture points (or *acu* points), which are the places where these *meridians* can be accessed to affect the life force running through them.

A good way to imagine this is to think of the *meridians* as underground railway lines, which lie beneath the skin, transporting a constant shuttle of 'trains' full of different types of energy around the body. The acupuncture points are like the stations, and are the places where it's possible to get onto the line and affect the ***Qi***. That's why we're so careful about identifying where a point is before inserting the needle: if you miss the station by a short distance you can't get on the train, as the rest of the track is underground, in a tunnel.

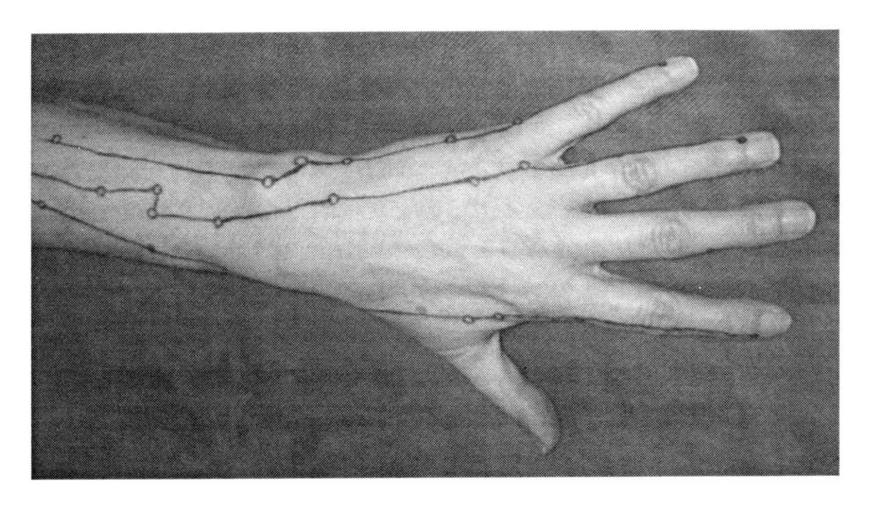

Meridians and points on the back of the hand and lower arm

Then, to get to the point…

Just shy of where two tendons meet,
Or quite deep in a cleft on the feet,
Search carefully, then
Decide on the ***men***—
Finding points is a feat, sweetly neat.

The *acu* points are tiny places where it's possible to connect with and affect the life force. Point location is a very important part of an acupuncturist's training. First we have to learn the anatomical locations: such as which bone a point is next to, or how many ***cun*** (anatomical Chinese inches) divide a point from a certain bodily 'landmark'.

Quite precise measurements and anatomical knowledge are required for the accurate location of many points. But when all the measuring is done, we have to feel, or palpate, for the precise position of the point. The exact place is often in a ***men***, which is Chinese for gate or doorway (meaning that this dip is viewed as an entrance to the point). It's usually a microscopic dip, and most acupuncturists become better at feeling these places with experience.

If your pain sears through each aching joint,
Don't take pills or with ointment, anoint.
Get a full diagnosis,
From your head to your toes-es:
Then the needle goes straight to the point.

Blood, the Substance

❧

Qi's upfront, while your *Blood's* undercover,
And they're matched, just like sister and brother.
Your ***Qi*** packs a punch,
While your *Blood's* made from lunch,
And each substance relies on the other.

In Chinese medicine we talk about the ***Qi*** and *Blood* as essential underlying foundations to good health. In the last section we discussed ***Qi,*** that mysterious, invisible life force that gives us 'oomph'. It's seen as the ***Yang***, or male of the two essential substances. *Blood* is the female, ***Yin*** counterpart.

As well as diagnosing problems with certain functions, your acupuncturist might decide that you are *Blood Deficient*, or that you have *Heat in the Blood* or *Blood Stagnation. Heat in the Blood* can lead to skin problems, and *Blood Stagnation* can cause painful periods, varicose veins or sharp pain in joints or muscles. In extreme cases *Stagnant Blood* can lead to clotting that causes a stroke.

There once was a hunter called Fudd,
Who, while chasing old Bugs, slipped on mud.
As he grabbed at that *wabbit*
He felt his leg stab—it
Was caused by a bruise (*Stagnant Blood*).

You've probably heard of Elmer Fudd, Bugs Bunny's great cartoon adversary, and I'm sure that, on occasions, Bugs has caused Elmer some acute incidents of *Blood Stagnation*. It can be a more long-term condition, too.

Deficiency is quite a problem in the Chinese view of blood pathology, which could mean that, despite a good, healthy diet, someone does not make enough blood to nourish the cells properly. In an extreme case this can lead to anaemia. Acupuncturists look at symptoms carefully, and a lack of hope or poor memory can be attributed to several different factors, one of which can be *Heart Blood Deficiency*.

There was a young lady whose *Heart*
Was deficient in *Blood*... so while smart,
She failed to remember
That date in December
When holidays frequently start.

Other *meridians* associated with *Blood* metabolism are the *Spleen*, *Kidneys*, *Stomach* and *Lungs*, and our task is to decide which one(s) to treat.

As usual, it is important to remember that when Chinese medicine describes a particular *meridian*, it does not necessarily equate fully with the Western medical description of the equivalent organ. For instance, if you've been a bit vague and ungrounded recently and your acupuncturist says they are treating your *Heart Blood*, don't worry, it's unlikely to mean you have a physical heart problem. Similarly, if you're feeling hopeless and depressed you might be treated for a deficiency of *Liver Blood*, but don't be concerned that you might have extreme liver disease: that's not what we're talking about.

Because women lose blood on a regular basis, with their periods, they are more prone to *Blood Deficiency* than men. It looks as though Elmer's daughter has different problems from her dad. Hmmm… I wonder if, in addition to having acupuncture treatment, it would help if she ate more meat, to feed her *Blood*… perhaps a little *wabbit*, for instance?

There was a young lady called Fudd,
Whose long periods had injured her *Blood.*
Since Doc Pins sent a shiver
To *Heart*, *Spleen* and *Liver.*
Her *Blood's* in full flow, but not flood.

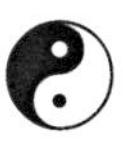

Is it Science?

Acupuncture has clear, defined rules,
Taught by masters and lately by schools:
Two thousand years' history
Reduces the mystery,
And separates wise ones from fools.

Acupuncture is based on Eastern science, which is different from Western science. This causes some people to suggest that, therefore, it is not science at all, as the implication is that only Western science counts.

However, Chinese medicine is extremely systemised and predates Western medicine by many centuries. The Chinese medical classics contain written history dating back more than 2,000 years, including diagnostic information and prescriptions. *The Nei Jing*, or *Yellow Emperor's Classic of Internal Medicine*, compiled between the second and third centuries BC, is a notable example and is still studied by students today. Ancient needles have also been found. There's a great history of ancient stone needles (yes, stone, yikes!) and gold and silver ones have been found which date back at least as far as the second century BC.

In ancient China, a doctor would have passed down acupuncture skills to his apprentices. In modern China, as in the West, acupuncture is taught in universities and other colleges and schools.

Nowadays there's a great deal of emphasis placed on research, and amongst the complementary medical systems, acupuncture has received a lot of attention. Once the difficulties of adequate double-blind systems are overcome, research frequently produces very favourable results for Chinese medicine against placebos and other treatments.

Arthritis, back pain and fertility are particularly well researched.

An Internet search on acupuncture and research will reveal the latest and longer-term results.

Researchers have long held a quest
For acu's success in the West.
Arthritis and pain,
And gynae all gain
Thumbs-up in a double-blind test.

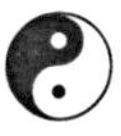

Diagnosis ~ What's All This About Tongues and Pulses?

Acupuncturists use all their skills,
Diagnosing and treating your ills.
They may look at your tongue,
Check your *Spleen* and your *Lung*,
And use needles instead of those pills.

Getting the correct diagnosis is a crucial part of traditional Chinese acupuncture. In order to decide which *meridians* (or channels of ***Qi*** energy) to treat, and which points to select on those pathways, your practitioner assesses as many aspects of you as possible, to get a complete understanding of the problems. It's like putting together a jigsaw puzzle: the more pieces we have, the better the picture. This involves gathering a case history, looking at your tongue and taking your pulses, as well as looking at physical things, such as complexion and physical structure.

The questioning part of the diagnosis usually starts with your immediate reasons for seeking treatment: probably physical or emotional problems. Additionally, we're interested to know anything you are willing to tell us about other symptoms, your medical history, and the usual systems checks, such as your digestion and sleep. Chinese medicine is based on a broader understanding of how things link together, as it is a truly holistic system, so we ask questions about heat tolerance, favourite climate, or whether the rain upsets you or affects your symptoms. And, of course, we're interested in your emotions and lifestyle.

In Chinese medicine's 2000-year written history, frequently a very specific symptom or feeling is written about, in the ancient classics, and as recently as in the past few hundred years. Such a description is often accompanied by suggested treatments, based on centuries of experience amongst Chinese doctors. As a result, we'll often ask patients about those odd things or tiny details that other practitioners may not find important.

In diagnosis you're asked to re-tell
Your medical history—as well
As what makes you feel good,
And you'll be understood
If you say that your pain hurts like hell.

We take pulses at the wrists to find out about the flow of ***Qi***. There are three pulse positions on each wrist, which give information about the health and balance of six different organs and functions… or even twelve if they are assessed in a certain way.

As in Western medicine, practitioners are interested in the simple pulse speed, but we also look for particular pulse qualities. These are described in certain terms, such as *Wiry*, which indicates pain or an issue on the *Liver* and *Gall Bladder* functions; *Slippery*, which indicates symptoms around the *Spleen* and *Stomach* functions or the presence of *Phlegm* in the body; *Thready*, which indicates a *Kidney* imbalance, or low energy; and so on. There are a variety of qualities, which are often present in different pulse positions on the same person. All of this adds to the information and gives more data for treatment planning.

Your treatment will often begin
With your pulses—too *Wiry* or *Thin*?
Are they *Slip'ry*, or *Knotted*?
This history is potted,
But Doc Pins will enquire within.

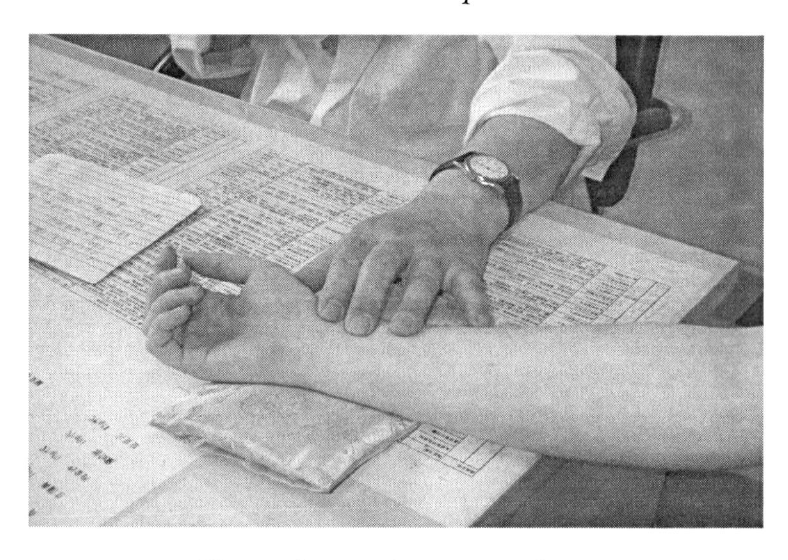

A Chinese doctor takes a patient's pulses

Another important feature of Chinese medical diagnosis is the examination of the tongue. We look at the colour of the tongue. From this we assess several things, including the quality and quantity of the *Blood*, and whether the patient is over-heating. We also look at any coating. This may indicate the presence of infection or a state of *Cold*, amongst other things. Cracks are also considered: for instance, cracks in the middle of the tongue can indicate a shortage of *Stomach* energy, which could indicate digestive problems.

There are many different possible configurations of information on the tongue, and each person's tongue has its own story to tell. One person's may show a picture that indicates a frail, weak body, while another may show that its owner is hot and impatient. The possibilities are almost endless, and there are entire books written on the subject.

If the cause of the illness, you're stalking,
Check the tongue for its signs, without baulking.
Is it red or quite pale?
Every crack tells a tale:
Though this tongue remains silent, it's talking.

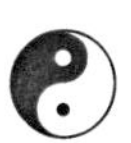

Syndromes, Organs and Meridians

Acupuncturists question your health
In some detail, which comes from a wealth
Of great knowledge from China:
No symptom is minor—
It's checked with bold questions and stealth.

Diagnosing according to the organs, functions and *meridians*, we put together all the information that has been gathered during the diagnosis, and arrange it into a diagnostic 'picture', according to which 'syndromes of imbalance' are showing most clearly. Usually this is a complicated picture, as by the time someone comes for treatment, their energy is generally quite a long way from the perfect balance they may have been lucky enough to have in early childhood.

The syndromes are particular patterns of disharmony within the organs, functions and *meridians*. For instance, a person with very depleted energy may have what is called ***Kidney Yin Xu*** (*yin shoo*). This is a weakness in the *Kidney* ***Yin*** energy, and it's a bit like having your background energy leaking out all the time, so you never really recover from your tiredness, whatever you may do to help yourself, such as sleeping and eating well.

Another person may have what is called ***Liver Qi*** *(chee)* ***Stagnation***. This is a situation in which the life force in the *Liver* function is not flowing freely, which may lead to digestive or menstrual problems, amongst other things. On an emotional level, it could also lead to anger or frustration, or a particular type of depression, in which the person sees no hope for the future.

Having decided on the syndromes of imbalance, we plan your treatment to help rebalance the energy in a particular group of organs or *meridians*.

There are many syndromes, with mysterious names like ***Spleen Qi Xu*** (*chee shoo*) and *Damp Heat in the Large Intestine*. This chapter gives just a glimpse of some of them, in relation to specific *meridians*. At the end of this section, there are also limericks on the three *meridians* that do not have their own syndromes. These are the *Three Heater*, ***Ren*** and ***Du*** *(doo) meridians*.

If you're tired, then perhaps there's ***Qi Xu***,
Or your *Kidney* is running low, too.
If you're angry, your *Liver*
Might just be the giver
Of, 'humph!' Or it might make you blue.

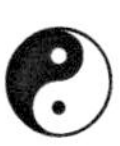

Can Acupuncture Help to Resolve Anger?

If your *Liver's* stagnated and tight,
As Ms Grumpy, you're ready to fight;
But when needled with skill
You can soften your will
And soon change to Ms Sweetnessandlight.

In Chinese medicine, the *Liver* function and *meridian* is understood to be responsible for the smooth flow of ***Qi*** (*chee/ life force*). The *Liver* is seen to have a much more comprehensive function than simply the physical one.

If someone's *Liver* ***Qi*** is not flowing properly, it is described as *Stagnant*. When this happens, the emotions are often affected as well as the physical body. If your acupuncturist has ever asked you, 'How's your temper at present?' having just had you describe something like your joint pains or headaches, the chances are they are diagnosing a certain amount of ***Liver Qi Stagnation*** in your system and would like to confirm how big a part of the overall picture this syndrome is at that particular time. If it is a significant feature that day, they will take steps to treat it.

At times like this, the chances are you will emerge from your treatment feeling calmer and less easily upset than before.

If you're angry and have a short fuse,
Acupuncture has points you can use.
Liver Qi that's stagnated
Is best abnegated
By needling right—that's good news!

After treatment, Mr or Ms Grumpy may not immediately change into Mr or Ms Sweetnessandlight, but, emotionally, you can feel considerably better quite quickly. This is good news for you and everyone around you!

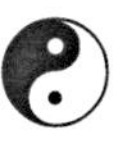

What Does the Spleen Have to Do with *Bounce*?

When your legs are so heavy and full,
And your head's filled with damp cotton wool,
If we tonify *Spleen*,
You could end up quite keen
To grab hold of the horns of the bull.

In Chinese medicine, the function of the *Spleen* controls the *Blood* and the transport of substances around the system. *Spleen* ***Qi*** is very important in the function of raising the energy within the body. If it's deficient, you can feel very tired or heavy, and possibly even suffer from a prolapse of the womb or bladder. This syndrome is called ***Spleen Qi Xu*** *(spleen chee shoo)*: literally, *Spleen* energy deficiency.

Spleen energy is also involved with the water metabolism, and we often diagnose a condition known as *Damp*. When likened to our immediate environment, you could see this rather as though the drainage in a house isn't working efficiently, and some damp has got stuck in the walls, which makes the whole house an unhealthy place to live.

Once we've diagnosed problems with the *Spleen* function, there are all sorts of treatment strategies. One very important acupuncture point on the *Spleen meridian* is translated from the Chinese as *Three Yin Crossing*. It also links with the *Kidney* and *Liver meridians*, which, along with the *Spleen*, are each described as ***Yin*** *meridians* on the lower part of the body.

"Exactly what is it you mean?
You're exhausted? And sinking? Come clean!
I'll just get Dr Pins
To tweak the *Three Yins*,
So your ***Qi*** can be raised by your *Spleen*.

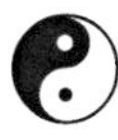

Nourishing the Kidneys For More Energy

If your battery pack's running low,
And your energy's running on 'slow',
We can charge you at 'trickle',
With nought but a prickle,
So your *Kidney* can get up and go.

In Chinese medicine, the *Kidney* function and *meridian* are viewed as the battery pack of the body, mind and spirit. For most people, from the age of about thirty-five (yes, that young!) *Kidney* energy begins to decline. When someone is more than casually short of this *Kidney* 'battery' energy, the syndrome of imbalance is known as ***Kidney Yin Xu*** or ***Kidney Yang Xu*** (pronounced *shoo*, and meaning deficiency). Symptoms can include tiredness and generally low energy, and can lead to many illnesses, including backache and urinary problems.

When treating either sub-set of ***Kidney Xu,*** we work hard to nourish the energy. However, we use points to fill up the deficiency gently, because it's unwise to treat the delicate *Kidney* function too heavily. This is similar to *trickle charging* your car battery if it's very low, as charging it too fast will ruin it. Consequently, if you have long-term illness or exhaustion, you will need regular treatment for a while.

Other symptoms of ***Kidney Xu*** include fear and disturbing or anxiety-filled dreams. We know that the adrenal glands, which produce the fear hormone, adrenaline, live on top of the kidneys. This hormone is released into the body during dangerous situations, to give us the instant energy boost to fight or run away (the fight or flight mechanism), so it's entirely logical that Chinese medicine associates the *Kidney meridian* and function with fear.

If your dreams are disturbing at night,
And you're anxious that all is not right,
Then your *Kidneys*, my dear,
Are too low, causing fear,
With adrenaline-filled fight or flight.

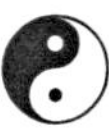

Lung Deals with Sadness and Sneezing

Do you cough with a permanent wheeze,
Or spend time with a spluttering sneeze?
Let's check on your tongue,
And then nourish your *Lung*,
'Cos such treatment's the key to bring ease.

As we know, the lung function/organ is responsible for taking in oxygen, which is transferred to the red blood cells and soon travels around the body, feeding each cell. It is also implicated in the protection from, or susceptibility to, coughs and colds. In Chinese medicine, the *Lung* includes the nose and throat, and the whole function provides a protective barrier to viruses. Consequently, if you catch every bug that goes around, we'll think about your *Lung* when making a diagnosis. It's also true that the *Lung* is deeply connected with the health of the skin and hair.

Less obvious to the Western way of thinking is the view that the *Lung* function is incredibly important in grief and sadness. If you're often sad or depressed we'll probably wonder about your *Lung*. (We may also think about your functions of *Heart*, *Pericardium*, and *Liver*.) If we decide that the *Lung* is a big player in your emotional issues there are several acupuncture points on this *meridian* that might be used. All points have names, translated from the Chinese, which often give a clue to their uses. Additionally, Western acupuncturists use a system of numbers on the *meridians*.

The *Lung meridian* has eleven points, from the top of the chest to the end of the thumb. *Lung 9*, a point on the wrist, is called *Great Abyss*, and one of its uses is to help people climb out of a deep hole of sadness. Sometimes this can give a noticeable lift to someone who is grieving, and it can also be used to help with depression.

If your feelings are sad and so dark,
And your life's full of grief and, well… stark,
Treatment won't go amiss
On *Lung 9, Great Abyss*,
To rekindle your life's missing spark.

Realistically, we need to remember that grief and depression do not simply disappear, even with acupuncture. These are deep-seated emotional conditions and need long-term, consistent treatment, whichever systems of medicine are chosen.

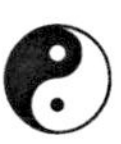

The Heart is Filled with Love as Well as Blood

The *Heart* governs *Blood* and the mind,
And it helps us be joyful and kind.
You could change palpitations
To good, good vibrations
And leave all your troubles behind.

The *Heart* and *Pericardium* (or *Heart Protector*) functions do look after our circulation and blood, and in Chinese medicine they also play a big part regarding emotions and certain kinds of anxiety.

There are quite a number of *Heart* function patterns or syndromes, ranging from ***Heart Yin Xu*** *(yin shoo)* and ***Heart Qi Xu*** *(chee shoo)* to the alarming-sounding *Heart Fire Blazing*, which is more dramatic and can result in more extreme symptoms of mental restlessness as well as physical symptoms, such as palpitations. It's important to note that these more intense syndromes are not very common, so if you are 'normally' anxious, you are very unlikely to be suffering from one of them.

The *Heart* is said to house the ***Shen***, or the *Spirit of the Mind*, and one of the principal acupuncture points for the treatment of physical or emotional shock is on the *Heart meridian*. It's called ***Shen Men***, which in Chinese means *Spirit Gate*.

The ancient Chinese viewed the organs/functions of the

body as a hierarchical government, with the *Heart* as emperor. In this system, the *Pericardium* is the emperor's bodyguard. Consequently, in acupuncture, a good deal of treatment for the *Heart* function is directed via the *Pericardium*.

Extreme anxiety is often diagnosed as emanating from the *Heart* function, though we also consider the *Kidney* function in this context. In fact, *Heart* and *Kidney* are frequently treated together, as issues with the *Kidney* function are often seen to lead to *Heart* function problems (heart and kidney problems have a relationship in Western medicine, too).

Sleep problems can also be related to the *Heart* or *Kidney* functions, especially if dreams are disturbing sleep.

Shen Men's a great point on the *Heart*
That helps settle when raw feelings smart.
If your dreams disturb sleep,
And emotions run deep,
Treating *Heart's* a great part of the start.

It is very important to note that when a practitioner of Chinese medicine diagnoses problems of the *Heart* function or *meridian* (from a **Chinese viewpoint**) they are not necessarily saying there is a problem with the physical heart, as it is viewed in Western medicine.

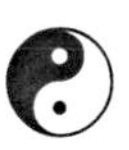

Do You Have the Gall to Act?

Fatty foods leave your innards appalled
When your *Gall Bladder's* feeling too galled—
So let's settle it down
With some needles (don't frown),
Then digest without feeling too mauled.

Like Western medicine, Chinese medicine sees that the *Gall Bladder* is very closely related to the *Liver* and is responsible for the metabolism of fatty foods. Consequently, poorly balanced *Gall Bladder* energy can lead to obesity, so treatment to adjust this might even help with slimming.

Additionally, it's seen as the function that has a great influence on the tendons and ligaments; so *Gall Bladder* points are often amongst those selected in the treatment of joint problems and sciatica. Along with the *Liver*, *Gall Bladder* issues are often diagnosed in instances of one-sided headaches and in sleeping problems.

Perhaps the aspect furthest from the Western perspective is the description of the *Gall Bladder* as the function most associated with decision-making. Again, this is very closely related to the *Liver's* mental function, which is the ability to plan, and it has a very important part to play in courage. Strong *Gall Bladder* energy equates to strong courage, while if you suffer from a lack of courage or self-determination, and if some of your other symptoms add up, we might decide you have ***Gall Bladder Xu*** *(shoo)*, or deficient *Gall Bladder* energy.

Your *Gall Bladder's* hold on the sinew,
On decisions and sleep will continue.
Great courage (not reckless)—
Without it, you're feckless—
And some careful adjustment could thin you.

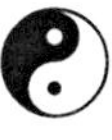

Can You Stomach It?

With this nausea, belching and hiccup
I feel kicked in the gut—what a stick-up!
To dissolve my sour frown,
Let's move ***Stomach Qi*** down
So my sense of well-being can pick up.

In Chinese medicine part of the *Stomach* function is described in ways that are obvious to Western thinking: 'rotting and ripening' and transforming food into life force (or ***Qi)***. It's also considered to be very important that the *Stomach* heats food to the optimum temperature for digestion, and there are several diagnoses and treatment strategies that deal with too much *Heat* or *Cold* in the *Stomach*.

Stomach Qi is said to have the quality of descending, and nausea and belching are signs that this is not happening properly, and the acupuncturist will take steps to correct it. Apart from people who regularly suffer this sort of discomfort, morning sickness in pregnancy also comes into the category of ***Rebellious Stomach Qi***, and because acupuncture has such a clear strategy for dealing with this problem, naturally, it's a great way to tackle it safely.

Stomach Qi is a very important factor in how energetic we feel, and someone who feels exhausted will often be treated on the *Stomach meridian*, as it is always possible to access '***Qi***

and Blood, (essential *substances*) via this function. One of the classic energising points is *Stomach 36* or ***Zu San Li*** (*Zoo San Lee*), translated as *Leg Three Miles*, which is a wonderful point for relieving exhaustion. Chinese people often say that this is the 'chicken soup' point, as they consider chicken soup (made with the addition of special herbs) to be one of the most nourishing foods. This is rather similar to the traditional Jewish view that chicken soup is a cure-all.

If your *Stomach* is prone to weak ***Qi***
Your hunger may drop a degree,
And perhaps you'll be tired
Until you've acquired
'Chicken Soup', which is called ***Zu San Li***.

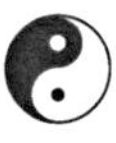

Do We Have to Talk About Bowels?

Your granny's advice in the home
Was don't sit on cool metal or stone,
For the cold will go in
To your bowel and begin
Diarrhoea with a moan and a groan.

In Chinese medicine, the large intestine, or colon, is viewed in a similar way to how it is in the West: it's the place where the body's waste products undergo a final reduction in water before being excreted. So most of the diagnostic patterns associated with this function have some reference to diarrhoea or constipation. In order to make a more accurate diagnosis, acupuncturists are not squeamish about the amount of detail they collect about the quality of the bowel movements, and there's even a special descriptive category called 'duck droppings' to describe how the excrement is in a certain case. You only have to walk around the edge of the duck pond in a city park to get the idea of what this is like!

Interestingly, Granny, in the limerick, was describing what Chinese medicine labels as *Cold Invading the Large Intestine*, which is an acute condition, possibly brought on by getting that lower part cold, just as Granny might have warned you. Whereas the 'duck droppings' problem would be labelled as *Large Intestine Cold* and would be a long-term, acute condition.

You could be forgiven for reading about these two syndromes and thinking they were the same thing, unless you were an acupuncturist looking at the whole patient 'picture', including a case history and tongue and pulse signs.

Because Chinese medicine defines many bowel issues as emanating from problems with other organs (often the *Spleen* and *Liver*), *Large Intestine* imbalances are not high on the list of diagnoses, or are often treated as being secondary to something else. But the *Large Intestine* does affect other things as well, and is even treated in certain cases of feverish colds and can be implicated in grief because it is strongly associated with the *Lung meridian.*

With sadness and fevers, the bowel
Can quite gruesomely cause you to howl—
There are duck droppings plopping,
Or guts that are stopping—
Large Intestine holds secrets quite foul.

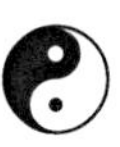

Small Intestine ~ Gutsy Stuff

If your taste for fast foods that are hot
Leads to guts with proverbial rot
And intestines so burning,
Or twisted and turning,
Some needles help loosen the knot.

The *Small Intestine* function can be damaged by regularly eating foods that are too hot or too cold and by obstruction of ***Qi*** (energy). For instance, *Full Heat in the Small Intestine* is a syndrome that describes fairly extreme and uncomfortable heat in the intestines, possibly associated with extreme thirst and even burning urine or blood in the urine. As with all the syndromes, these symptoms are not enough to decide a treatment plan, as the whole case picture must be taken into account.

Chinese medicine discusses the *Small Intestine* in terms of separating the pure fluids, which nourish the body, from the impure ones, which are eventually excreted. On the mental level it is also linked with clarity or restlessness. Mouth ulcers, poor hearing and even testicular pain can be seen as *Small Intestine* symptoms. However, it is often true that these symptoms are secondary to those of another function: perhaps the *Heart* or *Spleen*.

Small Intestine treats gut pain that's searing
And mouth ulcers, begging for clearing.
Then there's pain in the balls,
And confusion that calls,
"What d'yer say? Can you turn up my hearing?"

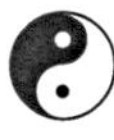

The Bladder Keeps the Body Pure

"Cystitis!" Repeating refrain,
So familiar, this thought in your brain—
Cold, Dampness below
Turned to *Heat*—now the flow
Is so urgent and burning—"Again!"

The *Bladder* function/*meridian* is particularly prone to problems resulting from *Damp*. You may think that's odd, as, surely, the bladder's entire job is to deal with water, so, of course it gets damp… But when we talk about *Damp* in the *Bladder*, we don't mean that the urine is damp (of course it's wet!) It's almost as though a slightly sticky sort of *Damp* has got into the very fabric of the bladder. (There's a chapter about *Pathogenic Factors*, which explains this in more detail.)

Damp gets in by rising up, either by a bug getting in through the urethra (the tube from the bladder to the outside world) or by getting too cold and damp, which leaves the body less able to fight off the bugs that would normally be killed by the naturally antiseptic nature of the urine.

Generally, this starts as a syndrome called *Damp-Cold in the Bladder*, which is recognisable as the need to urinate frequently and copiously. When this progresses to peeing small amounts of uncomfortably burning urine, the condition has changed to *Damp-Heat in the Bladder*. This happens for people who have a more ***Yang*** (or hot) body-type. You'll probably recognise this as cystitis. Post-menopausal women can be prone, since their ***Yin*** has depleted, making them hotter.

The bladder has a very important role in keeping the body fluids clean and healthy. Most imbalances of the *Bladder* function are treated with points on the *Bladder*, **Ren** and *Spleen meridians*, with back-up from points on other *meridians*, such as the ***Du*** (*doo*) and *Stomach* channels.

The *Bladder's* a reservoir (sort-a),
Which takes all the grubby old water;
Excretes from your body
Those fluids, most shoddy,
To clean up your act—or it oughta!

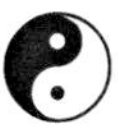

Heart Protector and Heating Engineer

Pericardium lives in the chest:
It's the sac round the *Heart* and the best
Kind of shield, for protection
From random infection
And emotions, when love's not so blessed.

There are two functions that are different from the ten organs represented by the main *meridians*. These are the *Pericardium* and the *Triple Burner*. Just to make matters more confusing, both go by more than one name.

The pericardium, or *Heart Protector*, is the membrane that surrounds the heart, and Chinese medicine sees it as the 'minister' that protects the *Heart* (which is described as the 'emperor' organ). Its main job is to protect the heart from harm or infection, so most inflammatory problems are intercepted by the pericardium before they reach the heart. It also has a connection with the blood, as does the heart. There are just a few *Pericardium* syndromes, and one of these, ***Pericardium Blood Xu*** (*shoo*), means it is deficient in *Blood*, and in addition to symptoms such as palpitations, insomnia and memory loss, there may be a tendency to being startled.

Chinese medicine is also very much in agreement with the popular idea of the heart's place in our emotional feelings. So it is very usual for an acupuncturist to treat on the *Pericardium meridian* if a person is feeling temporarily or long-term emotional. If someone feels unloved, it doesn't matter whether or not this is 'true': if the feeling is there it is often appropriate to treat the *Pericardium*. If someone is feeling a sense of loss, the acupuncturist might need to ask questions to establish whether to treat on the *Lung meridian* for one sort of grief and sadness, or on the *Pericardium* for a more *Heart*-type emotion.

The other function is the *Triple Burner*, also called the *Triple Warmer*, *Three Heater* and ***Sanjiao*** (pronounced *Sanjow*). It is involved in moving fluids around the system and also plays a big part in heating issues, so sore throats as well as fevers might be ascribed to an imbalance in this function. It sets and adjusts the thermostat and also balances the temperature in the different areas of the body as well as overall.

Your thermostat's carefully set
To balance your temperature, yet
If the ***Sanjiao*** is lacking
You might get a whacking
Great fever while bathed in hot sweat.

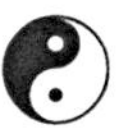

The *Ren* and *Du* Channels Make a Circuit

It sounds like a tiny, wee bird
With a tail sweetly turned-up—absurd—
I'll stop all this flannel:
The girliest channel,
Is ***Ren***, where the ***Yin*** is preferred.

As well as the twelve main *meridians*, there are eight extra ones. Of these, the two most commonly used are called ***Ren Mai*** (*Ren My*) and ***Du Mai*** (*Doo My*). Whereas the organs (*Heart*, *Stomach*, *Kidney* etc) have a *meridian* or channel on each side of the body, the ***Ren*** and ***Du*** channels are central, so each has only one line.

The ***Ren*** channel, also called the *Conception Vessel*, is the most ***Yin***, or female, of all the *meridians* and is important in the treatment of gynaecological problems. Amongst other things, it's also employed in urinary disorders, tight chest, digestive dysfunction and exhaustion. It travels centrally up the front of the body.

The ***Du*** channel, also called the *Governor Vessel*, is the most ***Yang***, or male, *meridian*. It's used is some situations of dizziness, depression, fever and manic behaviour and when the back is weak. It's also used with prolapses, as it strengthens and pulls ***Qi*** (*life force*) upwards. As with the ***Ren Mai***, this *meridian* runs centrally on the body, this time mainly on the back, starting at the base of the coccyx.

Together, these two central *meridians* make a complete circuit around the trunk of the body and the head.

It starts where the butt shows a crack,
To rise, centrally, straight up your back.
If you're manic or slow,
Or some fever's aglow,
Then the ***Du Mai*** brings ***Yang*** back on track.

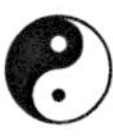

Yin and Yang ~ Life's Balancing Foundation

ஃ

Yin and ***Yang*** are the basis of life:
They oppose (but in balance, not strife).
Yin is *substance*, ***Yang's Qi***;
And ***Yin's*** 'she', to ***Yang's*** 'he'—
They're the perfect team: husband and wife.

'Yin and Yang' is a term that has made its way into our English vocabulary. Sometimes we say things like, "It's all about ***Yin*** and ***Yang***", with a good understanding about it, but sometimes people just say it because it has a certain oriental 'cool' to it in these days when acupuncture and films about martial arts are so popular.

In Chinese philosophy ***Yin*** and ***Yang*** are the twin foundations of life: the light and shade, which make everything possible because they balance and counterbalance each other. ***Yin*** is the feminine part of that foundation and ***Yang*** is the masculine. Both are equally important, and are seen as the essential opposites: ***Yin*** is the principle behind night, while the ***Yang*** force is most active in the day. ***Yin*** is to the moon what ***Yang*** is to the sun; ***Yin*** is cold, ***Yang*** hot, and so on.

The list is endless, and everything is a mix of both principles, so, for instance, while the moon is categorised under the influence of ***Yin,*** it is also made up of a perfect balance of ***Yin*** and ***Yang***, in which ***Yin*** predominates slightly. While a man is seen as ***Yang***, he is also considered to be a perfect combination of ***Yin*** and ***Yang***, with enough emphasis on the ***Yang*** side of things for him to be recognisably a man in body and attitude.

In Chinese medicine, ***Yin*** and ***Yang*** are seen as an essential mixing balance within the body-mind-spirit. Half of the *meridians* that are treated with acupuncture are predominantly ***Yin***, while the others are predominantly ***Yang***.

Yin relates to the darkness and moon,
While she's cool and does nothing too soon.
She's the feminine force—
Controls childbirth, of course—
And lives deep, in the safest cocoon.

Yin is the dark, introspective part of life's energy. As well as governing the night, the moon and cold, it (she) governs slowness, stillness and things that descend. In Chinese medicine, ***Yin*** is responsible for the *Blood* and fluids: for the substance of the body. As the feminine principle, it is heavily responsible for the health of female things, like menstruation and pregnancy.

If you easily become dehydrated or tired, or are suffering from menopause or period problems, we'll certainly be looking to see what's happening to your ***Yin*** organs, such as *Kidney*, *Spleen* and *Liver*. The others are *Lung* and *Heart*; and the *Pericardium* function, and the extra *meridian*, ***Ren*** (or

Conception Vessel) also belong to ***Yin***.

Yang is brightness and outward-going. As well as day and heat, it (he) is also in charge of movement, speed and things that ascend. In Chinese medicine, the ***Qi*** (*life force*) is the domain of ***Yang:*** that's the life energy, as opposed to the fluids/substance of life that are ***Yin's*** responsibility.

So, if you get overheated or agitated in an excess-energy way, we'll want to assess what is happening to your ***Yang*** energy. The primarily ***Yang*** organs are *Small Intestine, Bladder, Stomach, Large Intestine* and *Gall Bladder*, while the *Three Heater* (or ***Sanjiao***) function and the ***Du*** *meridian* (or *Governor Vessel*) are also ***Yang***.

Yang's so bright, like the sun and the day;
Houses ***Qi***, to support work and play.
While outward and male;
This guy's hot and not pale,
And prepared to put all on display.

Of course, just as the whole of life is a complex mix and balance of ***Yin*** and ***Yang***, so is every person who has acupuncture treatment. Consequently the causes behind illness will be a mixture of ***Yin*** and ***Yang***-related problems, and that's where your acupuncturist's diagnostic skill comes in.

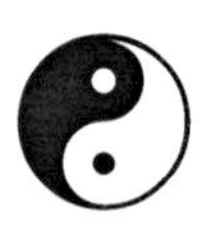

The Five Elements

Wood flows into *Fire*: *Fire* to *Earth*,
Then to *Metal*, then *Water* gives birth
Back to *Wood*, in the circuit:
With know-how to work it,
This theory is loaded with worth.

Chinese philosophy has one more element than the Western version. *Fire*, *Earth* and *Water* all sound familiar to the Western ear, but where does *Metal* fit in… and *Wood*, come to that? *Metal* represents the mineral element, and is the equivalent to air in Western thought.* *Wood* is the extra one, the element representing growing things, or the plant kingdom.

In the theory of *Five Elements*, all five co-exist in a continuously self-nourishing cycle. There is a particular sequence to this cycle, as each element gives birth to and nourishes the next one. As in the first limerick in this section, the circle is: *Wood>Fire>Earth>Metal>Water>Wood* etc., though, of course, the cycle can begin with any one element. Some of these 'mother-child' relationships are more obvious than others. We can all understand easily why *Wood* would feed *Fire*, and we can see that *Fire* feeds *Earth*, in that ash becomes a very important component of earth and a bush fire cleanses and regenerates the life-sustaining properties of the earth. *Earth* can be seen as the mother of *Metal*, in that pockets of minerals are held within the 'womb' of the earth, and Metal feeds Water, in that de-mineralised water is pretty much 'dead' water. And, finally, without water, wood/plants would not be able to grow.

Going round in a circle I found
That my circular trail would abound
With continuous curves,
Making long, drawn-out swerves,
Till I started again… going round…

In acupuncture theory, each *meridian* belongs to a particular element, and each element has many relationships to substances and more subtle things, such as the senses. For instance, the *Wood* element embraces the *Liver* and *Gall Bladder meridians* and in diagnosis it is related to the colour green, so if a person's face has a slightly greenish hue, the practitioner will check to see how big an impact the *Liver* and *Gall Bladder* have in the person's imbalance or disease. When you think about it, even in Western medicine, a greenish complexion is associated with a livery or bilious condition. While Chinese medicine takes this into consideration, it also takes the skill of observation further.

In diagnosis, each element is also associated with a particular odour, sound and emotion. For instance, if we notice that a scent of new ironing accompanies a patient into the room, we might be alerted to look for other signs that this person has an imbalance in the *Fire* element, as the particular aroma associated with *Fire* is 'scorched'. In Western medicine, traditionally, doctors would use the sense of smell amongst other skills, to assess the patient, but nowadays, machines and lab tests have left behind these more human skills of diagnosis.

I won't go into details about all the ways we assess, but within the *Five Element* picture, we look for anything that seems to point in a particular direction. The patient's emotional character is particularly relevant. There are other factors, too, such as their preferred tastes or the locations of symptoms within the body: for instance having weak muscles or frequent stomach problems might lead us to think about the *Earth* element.

In Chinese medicine, each element within a person should be in balance, as this means the person's body works in harmony. However, according to *Five Element* theory, most people have a dominant element, which is part of what makes them the particular sort of individual they are. When this predisposition becomes exaggerated, however, it can lead to illness, and rebalancing with the help of acupuncture treatment is a very good plan.

When we're fit, the *Five Elements* match,
But in sickness, they squabble and scratch,
Till we're sad or annoyed,
And good health is destroyed...
To re-build will need more than a patch.

* *Metal* is equivalent to air? Yes, and strange though it may sound, one way to get your head around this concept is to think about the chemical elements in air, which could, at a pinch, be seen as minerals. In acupuncture the *Metal* element is very connected with air and breath, as one of the *Metal* organs is *Lung*.

The Wood Element

Creatively full of desire—
Your ideas could be magic or dire!
You'll have qualities spanning
From arts to good planning.
If you're patient, your work will inspire.

Creativity and forward planning are big characteristics of the '*Wood* person'. We all have this part to our nature, but a predominantly *Wood*-type character might be fantastically arty or able at making plans… or they might be hopelessly inflexible and unable to change a plan to save their life.

An unfortunate side of this creative element is that when frustrated, the creativity can turn to grumpiness or anger. The classic 'artistic temperament' contains features that relate to the *Wood* element.

Each element governs certain bodily components, and *Wood* is particularly associated with the tendons and ligaments, and also with the eyes and eyesight. There's even a specific 'sound' that goes with each element, and it may not surprise you to know that for *Wood* it's the sound of shouting—possibly not literal shouting, but an assertive speaking voice. If you've ever puzzled over why someone seems to 'broadcast' to the neighbourhood each time they open their mouth, maybe they have an issue with their *Wood* element.

As I mentioned in the introduction to this section, the *meridians*/organs that belong to the *Wood* element are the *Liver* and *Gall Bladder*. This does not necessarily mean a *Wood*-type of person will have gallstones or liver problems, but it's a possibility. There are all sorts of reasons that explain why the physical symptoms may or may not relate to the organs of the person's most 'personal' element, and there are good books written on the subject.

You're cross and creative by turns,
With a temper so grumpy, it burns.
You might shout when you speak
Or have tendons that creak.
Wood learns, or dismissively spurns.

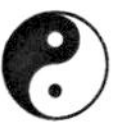

The Fire Element

You sweetheart, you dear, lovely child,
Your manners and bearing are mild,
But your temper can flare-up,
Or you're sad, so please cheer-up,
Then your laughter will drive us all wild!

The '*Fire* person' probably has big issues around love and laughter. Their social skills might be great, or they could be introverted… or a bit of both. We all know about the traditional clown character, who makes everyone laugh in the circus ring or on the stage and then goes home full of sadness... or the person who is the life and soul of the party, yet prone to bouts of depression.

The insecurity and vulnerability of the very '*Fiery*' person is an area a *Five Element* acupuncturist will notice and work on. As with all the other elements, the *Fire* can be brought back, nearer to balance. The *Fire* person will probably always be '*Fiery*', but with good acupuncture treatment they can become friendly, warm *Fire*.

The *Fire* organs are the *Heart* and *Small Intestine*, and there are two functions: the *Pericardium* is the protective sac around the *Heart* and the *Triple Burner* (or ***Sanjiao*** *[sanjow]*) is the heating engineer in the body-mind-spirit.

While the *Fire* temper can flare up, like the flames in a fire, it also dies down equally fast, unlike the resentful '*Woody*' temper or the critical *Metal* temper.

In dysfunction, our *Fire* friends dissolve
Into states that quite often involve
Thoughts like… "Nobody loves me,
And everyone shoves me
Aside" … which are hard to resolve.

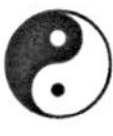

The Earth Element

A home-making person, is *Earth*—
So provisions won't run into dearth.
There'll be food in your tumsy,
With a home-loving mumsey:
So beware... an expansion of girth!

Home's an important place for the *Earth* person… or not, depending on how healthy their *Earth* is. You have probably met plenty of *Earth* people who are great hosts and make you feel welcome with delicious little snacks or lovely meals. Some *Earth* people make great restaurateurs, as they satisfy their desire to feed the world.

The *Earth* element's associated organs are the *Stomach* and *Spleen*, so an out of balance *Earth* element causes disturbance in the digestion. The main bodily components associated are the muscles, so a tendency towards being overweight or skinny can both be problems associated with *Earth*. But don't forget, we'll be looking for and weighing up all sorts of different signs and associations before labelling someone as *Earth*. There's an associated colour, too: yellow.

The emotion associated with the *Earth* element is sympathy, and *Earth* people do often exhibit neediness or can even be labelled as hypochondriacs, but they can also be wonderfully sympathetic towards others. As with the other elements, each *Earth* person is unique.

You poor thing, does your body feel rough,
With some aching and sickness, and stuff?
Facing bad diarrhoea,
You look yellow, my dear.
Is my sympathy touching enough?

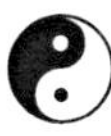

The Metal Element

Your standards are higher than high,
And you're truthful (why **would** people lie?)
Though you're open to reason,
To betray you is treason—
But your spirit is strong and won't die.

Classically, the *Metal* person has very high (or, more unusually, very low standards) depending on many things. They'll often have strong feelings about the spirit: they may have religious views, or maybe they'll be an atheist, or perhaps someone who likes to meditate. Truth is another important issue.

A *Metal*-type person who is in pretty good emotional health is often someone who does a job carefully and who you would automatically trust to be responsible and honourable.

Along with these thoughts and abilities goes a desire to be perfect, or a feeling of not being good enough, which can be very hard work for them (and those around them… it can even be difficult to get some *Metal* people to accept praise!) So it figures that the associated emotion is grief.

The organs associated with the *Metal* element are the *Lungs* and *Large Intestine*, and the skin is also very important. As each element has a colour associated with it, the one for *Metal* is white.

If your *Lung* pulse is weak and quite low,
You may think, "Am I good enough? No!"
While your feelings of grief
Won't exactly be brief...
Holy Crow, you've an eerie white glow!

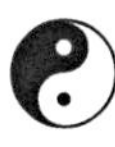

The Water Element

When *Watery* feelings run deep,
You'll find your own counsel to keep.
As you bubble along
With a will that is strong,
Have no fear, but please look where you leap.

Like a river or stream, *Water* can be the hardest element to get a hold of or understand—it just runs through your fingers or your mind.

Fear is the emotion associated with *Water*, and many people who have this element out of balance will exhibit a lot of fear. '*Watery*' people often look at life from a perspective of anxiety, and one of the tasks of the acupuncturist is to help them get this fear more under control.

However, there are some people who have *Water* as their dominant element, and fear appears to be lacking in a rather alarming way. For these people, the adrenaline rush may be more important than avoiding danger. Have you ever wondered what drives those extreme sports fanatics?

The associated organs are the *Kidneys* and *Bladder*, which makes sense of the fear, or the lack of it, as the adrenal glands live on top of the kidneys and govern the mechanism known as 'fight or flight'... in other words, in the face of danger people either stand and fight or run away.

I watched Evil Knievel perform…
As the stunt-rider revved up a storm,
Did adrenaline 'plus'
For jumping that bus
Make danger feel more like the norm?

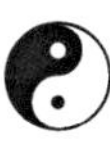

The Shaoyang Level ~ When Illness Gets Stuck

When disease is half out and half in,
We will surely decide to begin
With ***Shaoyang*** to remove
All the dross, and improve
Deeper health, which lies dormant within.

Chinese medicine recognises that some illnesses get trapped inside the body. This explains those situations when someone says, 'I've never been the same since I had that very bad virus that turned into a chest infection', or 'Since I had glandular fever I haven't regained my full health.' A person might even have been diagnosed with chronic fatigue syndrome (ME). There are many variations on this theme. For instance, often an anaesthetic or a course or two of antibiotics can be part of the picture.

Whatever the cause, we see it as a situation in which disease or its debris has become stuck, and so has the effect of blocking the body's clean-up mechanism and immune function.

One way acupuncturists describe what happens when you take antibiotics is this: you are upstairs and you hear burglars in the sitting room (the burglars are the illness or infection), so you go downstairs and shoot the burglars (you take antibiotics to kill the infection). Then you have the problem of the burglars' bodies in your sitting room. It may be difficult to remove them and they may start to decay, making the house an unhealthy and less pleasant place to live (the debris from the dead bacteria lodges in your system and clogs it up, which affects your health and immunity). So you need a special tool to flush out the dead bodies.

That's where acupuncture comes in. We work on what we call the ***Shaoyang*** *(show-yang)* level, which is where things get stuck half way out and half way in the body. We use certain acupuncture points to clear out the old debris, and so allow the body to function well once again.

What's that noise in the night, well, hell, dang!
It's burglars. I'll shoot 'em all: BANG!
Now the room's out of use,
Jammed with bodies, so puce.
I'd better clear up with ***Shaoyang***.

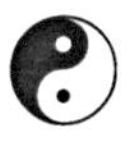

Pathogenic Factors Slow Down Recovery

If your illness has lasted for ages,
And your remedies run on for pages,
You might suffer a pathogen,
Or react to an allergen,
Chinese medicine can help you, in stages.

Chinese medicine has a unique take on why some illnesses occur. There is a long-held understanding that external factors invade or internal factors get stuck in the body if the natural protective layer and immunity are not up and running properly. These forces can seriously slow down recovery, and are called *Pathogenic Factors*. To the Western ear some of them sound rather like a weather forecast, with a 'yuk factor' thrown in for good measure!

The commonly diagnosed invading factors are: *Wind*, *Cold*, *Heat*, *Dryness*, *Damp* and *Phlegm* (yes, *Phlegm's* the non-weather report, yukky one…)

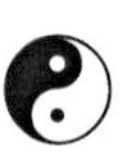

Wind

In your low, plunging neckline (so cool),
During winter, you may play the fool.
Would your granny approve?
Does your neck hurt to move?
There's a point that will help you... *Wind Pool.*

Wind is the first factor to consider, as this can bring other factors (*Cold*, *Heat*, *Dryness* or *Damp*) into the body with it.

External *Wind* is often deemed to have invaded the body through the neck and shoulders when they haven't been properly protected against outside forces. The chilling truth is that if your granny ever told you to wear a scarf she was probably right! Chinese people (and acupuncturists) are dead keen on wearing enough clothes to protect this vulnerable part of the body.

According to Chinese medicine, as well as the upper shoulder region, a very vulnerable place is the back of the neck, just under the skull. One of the best acupuncture points to eliminate *Wind* invasion is just there, and is called *Wind Pool* (**Feng Chi**).

As well as causing obvious symptoms, like stiff neck, *Wind* is also seen as an *internal* factor involved in the sorts of illnesses that cause shaking, such as Parkinson's disease, and also in strokes.

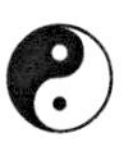

Cold

If you dread every temperature drop,
When your pulse nearly slows to a stop,
And with winter's cold fingers,
The ice in you lingers,
Have needles with moxa on top.

Cold is a frequent invader. Many people feel almost permanently cold, and for some it can feel as though it's deep in the bones: it can take months to warm up, even in summer.

If you're a *Pathogenically Cold* person, you may look at others who are wearing skimpy tops, and inwardly shiver, and you may dread winter. Have you ever wondered if you're a wimp, or whether it's in your imagination? Well, it's real, and some consistent acupuncture treatment that includes points which are known to expel *Cold* can make a big difference. We might also use ***moxibustion*** (or ***moxa***) on you, which is a treatment in which dried herbs are burned on or near the body to help warm you through to a deep level.

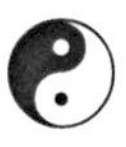

Heat

Oh wow, you're so gorgeous, you're hot,
But that T-shirt's most certainly not!
I just cannot believe
That your coolest shirt sleeve
Is your choice when hot summer it's not!

The opposite of the *Pathogenically Cold* person is the *Hot* one. If you're the person in the skimpy top or T-shirt in the dead of winter, you probably break out in sweat just thinking about that *Cold* person all wrapped up in their winter woollies – indoors!

An acupuncturist will ask you questions about your reaction to different temperatures and climates, and if we identify *Pathogenic Heat* as a problem we'll include points in your treatment plan that are known to dispel extra *Heat*. Don't worry, though, this won't make you a *Cold* person, but it will help you to overcome those uncomfortable times when you overheat.

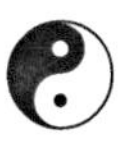

Dryness

With *Dryness*, you're parched, and your skin
Can be papery, dried-up and thin.
And playing the stud,
Can injure your *Blood*.
For treatment, we'll nourish your ***Yin***.

Dryness is a *Pathogenic Factor* that doesn't affect us very much in Britain, at least not externally, as drying, heat-carrying winds don't really blow in from the desert here! However, internal *Dryness* is something that can affect us.

Acupuncturists explain that as we age (from about thirty-five onwards) we lose some of our ***Yin*** energy. We are all made of a combination of ***Yin*** and ***Yang***, and Chinese medicine describes ***Yin*** as the energy that helps our bodies to retain the correct balance of moisture. So, because we have less ***Yin*** as we get older, we become *Dryer*. This means we can become thirsty more easily, and our skin and secretions start to dry out. Even our *Blood* becomes thicker and stickier, which affects how well our cells are nourished.

Apart from ageing, other things can deplete our ***Yin***, such as smoking, alcohol and eating too much of certain types of foods. For men, too much sex can deplete the ***Yin***, especially as they age, so Chinese medicine recommends caution in this department, too… (but not abstinence!)

Many acupuncture treatments will include points to help counteract dryness. We describe these points as ones that ***Nourish the Yin***.

Damp

Does that heaviness make you less keen
To move on? ("I wish... speedy and lean!")
To get *Dampness* to drain,
The best treatment, in main,
Should be points chosen largely on *Spleen*.

Pathogenic Damp can make you feel sluggish, tired and heavy. It can also mean that you hold on to a little more weight than is ideal… or a lot more if the *Damp* is long-term. Having internal *Damp* can also make you more susceptible to climatic damp, so, people with *Damp* often feel worse in wet or humid weather.

If we identify this factor as a problem, we'll include *Damp-dispelling* acupuncture points in your treatments, and some of the most frequently used ones are on the *Spleen meridian.* Depending on your diagnosis, ***moxa*** may also be used to help drive *Damp* out of your body.

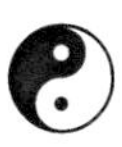

Phlegm

What's that you just said to me, Steph?
I'm not really substantially deaf—
But this gunk in my ears
Will reduce me to tears.
Yukky *Phlegm's* such a deafly *PF!**

Phlegm sounds truly yuk, doesn't it? It can sometimes be seen as an extension of *Damp*… a sort of thickening of *Dampness* that is stuck in the body. It can also be just what it sounds like: mucusy, sinusy problems, and sometimes issues with things like blocked tubes in the ears. This can be a problem with children who routinely have blocked ears or glue ear. (So it would be good to consider acupuncture if your child is heading towards having ear grommets fitted.)

We also diagnose something called *Insubstantial Phlegm*, which is *Phlegm* that has been driven deep into the system and is difficult to identify because it is not visible. We often consider this as a possibility in 'mysterious' diseases such as MS and chronic fatigue syndrome (ME).

As with all *Pathogenic Factors** (or *PFs*), *Phlegm* will slow down any recovery. Whether or not *Phlegm* is visible, if we identify that you have it, we'll be keen to help you to clear it.

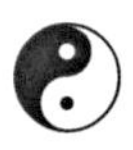

Interlude...

Today I'll learn acu Chinese—
Words for needle, intestine and wheeze:
I'll learn "How do you do?"
And Shi down to Xu,
And that Phlegm-forming stuff—is that Qi-z?

Few Western-trained acupuncturists speak Mandarin Chinese, but most have to learn odd little bits, mainly to do with acupuncture terminology. So, learning words such as Xu (shoo), which means deficiency, and Shi (shuh) for excess, is normal. Those of us who are fortunate enough to take our Western-based training further, spending some time in acupuncture schools or hospitals in China, might also learn a few polite phrases for addressing patients. Most of us can at least manage "Ni hau" (nee how), which means, "Hello!"

Of course the last line of the limerick is a travesty of Chinese... 'Qi' (chee) is one of the most common terms, as it is the Chinese word for life force, and there really is no accurate English equivalent. Chinese medicine has a lot of theory about diet and health, and there's a whole list of Phlegm-forming foods, including bananas, peanuts and cheese.

Same Symptom ~ Different Treatment?

Be it backache, damned hormones, rough skin,
Bad migraines, or troubles within—
Whatever condition,
Doc Pins' position
Is make a fresh plan and begin.

Chinese medical diagnosis is elegant in its complexity. One of its beauties is that we diagnose each person as a unique individual. Consequently, the acupuncturist views no one as 'a case of arthritis' or 'a skin problem'. Yes, the person may have arthritis or a skin condition, but during the diagnosis we'll focus on evaluating which patterns of disharmony within each particular person's body-mind-spirit are causing the symptoms.

For instance, no one is seen as just 'a headache'! We'll evaluate the patient who has headaches to find out what is causing the pain in terms of a complex and interwoven number of factors. Throughout the diagnosis, we may build a picture of a particular person, which shows that their headaches are across the forehead, are worse in hot, humid weather, and that that person also has a weight issue and gets over-heated very easily. Then we may see another 'headache person', whose symptoms are on one side of the head and are triggered when the person is cold or hungry or tired, or when they've had a drink or two. This is a tiny example of a few of the possibilities for diagnosis of just one symptom.

Whether the problem is headaches, post-operative trauma, menstrual irregularity or any number of other things, we put together as much information as possible, in order to increase the accuracy of the treatment plan. And to make this picture even more accurate, we consider as much other information as possible about that person.

So two 'headache' friends who have a chat about their respective acupuncture treatments may be quite surprised to find that they have needles placed in different points on their bodies.

Each person has symptoms distinct
(Whether complex, or neatly succinct),
So Doc Pins has the task
To look, listen and ask,
Then decide how your problems are linked.

The rest of this chapter will give you an idea of diverse treatment strategies for some common symptoms. If something you suffer from is not included, don't worry, these are just examples. In Chinese medicine there is a way to diagnose each different pattern or symptom 'picture'.

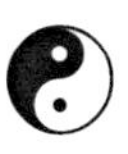

Colds and Flu Come in Different Varieties

If your nose is all 'snivel and run',
And you long for a life in the sun,
With a pin in *Lung 7*,
Though still not in heaven,
You're likely to find things more fun.

You may think that a cold is a cold, is a cold. But we divide the common cold into different types, depending on the symptoms. Mostly, we start by diagnosing what we call an invasion by *Wind*. This is what breaks through the protective layer that should act as a barrier to *bugs*. *Wind* carries with it either *Cold* or *Heat*, depending on circumstances and personal weakness. For instance, whatever type of virus is around at the time, some people will always seem to get a sore throat, whereas other people will get a head cold that goes to the chest, and so on.

Snivelly colds are usually diagnosed as deriving from an invasion of *Wind-Cold*, whereas ones with a sore throat or temperature are often described as being triggered by *Wind-Heat* (and are typical of summer colds).

One of the points on the *Lung meridian*, *Lung 7*, is frequently chosen as part of the treatment for a *Wind-Cold* invasion. It's called ***Lie Que*** *(lee kway)* or *Broken Sequence*. When sweating, *Heat* or a sore throat is a symptom, it's quite usual to include in the treatment a point from the ***Sanjiao*** *meridian* (pronounced *san-jow*). This is one of the stranger-sounding *meridians*.

There isn't really an equivalent in the English language, and it doesn't correspond to an organ. It's also known as the *Triple Burner meridian*, as it's used to help regulate the body's heating mechanism.

When you catch a rough cold from *Wind-Heat*,
The symptoms could make your voice bleat.
As your throat's red and sore,
And you sweat from each pore,
Treating ***Sanjiao***, your *Heat* will retreat.

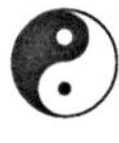

Different Headache ~ Different Treatment

Slicing pain to the side of my head—
Now my eye's sharply stabbed, in its stead.
I feel terribly queasy—
My stomach's uneasy—
I've fled to the dark of my bed.

From the perspective of Chinese medicine, every headache is different. While we assess each individual occurrence in its own right, there are some general categories, which help us to diagnose accurately.

Two of the key areas of assessment are the position of the headache and how the pain or ache feels. For instance, a stabbing headache may be caused by *Blood Stagnation*. In other words, the blood is not flowing well enough and becomes too thick and sticky, so not enough oxygen is carried to the head. A muzzy headache that makes you feel as though your head is wrapped in a damp towel will probably be associated with the *Spleen* and *Stomach* and internal *Damp*.

Areas of the head are associated with different *meridians* or functions. For instance a *Liver* imbalance can cause a headache in the middle of the crown of the head. Chinese terms for pairs of *meridians* are often used to describe some of the other types. A ***Yangming*** headache is associated with an imbalance of the *Stomach* or *Large Intestine meridian*, so once we identify this pattern, we'll decide on a treatment accordingly, probably on one or both of these *meridians*. The

Shaoyang *(show-yang)* pairs the *Gall Bladder* and ***Sanjiao*** (*Triple Burner*) *meridians*, and a ***Taiyang*** *(tie-yang)* headache refers to one that hurts on the *Bladder meridian* and is also associated with an imbalance in the *Small Intestine* function.

Yangming makes your forehead like lead,
While ***Shaoyang*** grabs your temples instead.
Taiyang aches like heck
In the back of your neck,
And *Liver* sits high on your head.

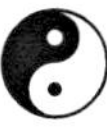

Giving Injuries a Sporting Chance

A young man from near Neasden loved sport:
Now he sports for his sport a support.
Chinese medicine could free
Nobby's sore, bashed-up knee—
What a sporting good sort of a thought!

Sports injuries can happen to anyone: from the super-fit to the wannabe fit. So, as with treatment for other problems, we assess sports injuries differently on different people.

Because Chinese medicine is based on a truly holistic system of diagnosis, it is very likely that if you visit an acupuncturist when you have a sports injury, we'll ask you questions about your general health and check your tongue and pulses, in addition to asking about the injury itself.

This is great, as your overall health is likely to benefit as well as the damaged part. You could end up feeling better than you have done for years, simply because you sprained your shoulder whilst skiing and had some acupuncture treatments to help with the pain.

If you visit an acupuncturist for a one-off emergency treatment following an injury and you are in relatively good health, you may possibly just receive treatment to the local area.

Work on the damaged area could include treatment with acupuncture needles, ***moxibustion*** or *cupping*. If your practitioner is trained in the use of Chinese herbal medicine, you may also be given some spray or lotion to help with sprains or bruising.

Young Elizabeth damaged her wrist,
(Squished at squash... hit too hard... wished she'd missed!)
Then she let out a yelp,
Called Doc Pins for some help...
And the gist? "Help this twist to desist!"

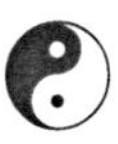

Burning the Midnight Oil

If you can't get your jolly old head
Around sleeping, when tucked up in bed,
Acupuncture can calm
Swirling thoughts, like a balm—
Then your head can go z-z-z-zed.

Sleeping difficulties can have enormously negative effects on our health in general; so Chinese medicine takes a serious view of this problem. During the diagnosis we'll set about deciding which organ (or function) imbalances are most fundamental in causing the patient's problems. For instance, Chinese medical knowledge states that, in addition to its important role in *Blood* metabolism and detoxification, the *Liver* function is responsible for the smooth flow of ***Qi*** (*chee, life force*). This smooth flow helps us to feel calm and relaxed. Consequently, if the *Liver* function is impaired and the ***Qi*** is not flowing smoothly we may feel hyperactive or 'wired'. For various reasons, this is likely to become exaggerated at night and can be a major cause of sleeping problems.

However, not all insomnia is caused by *Liver* function imbalance. For instance, the *Heart Spirit*, or ***Shen*** is responsible for keeping the mind calm. So when someone is traumatised or uneasy for emotional reasons, we may diagnose ***Shen*** disturbance. This can also lead to sleeping issues, as the mind is too bothered to settle down.

Another background cause could be a depletion of ***Kidney Qi***. In Chinese medicine the *Kidney* function is seen as the body's battery pack, so it's important to keep this energy topped-up. If we become very depleted it's possible to get too tired to sleep. Have you ever experienced this? You're exhausted, but somehow it's gone beyond the point where you can simply go to sleep to top-up on energy, so it becomes a vicious circle. Actually, at this point it's likely that we'll diagnose a more complex syndrome, such as depleted ***Kidney Qi*** affecting the ***Shen*** (*Heart spirit*) or the ***Liver Qi***. When out of harmony, the *Heart* and *Kidney* can cause anxiety, so they are often treated together when someone is experiencing that particular sort of disturbance.

Fortunately, all these diagnoses lead to a variety of treatment strategies, though it's fair to say that if you have long-term insomnia it may take a while to bring your sleeping pattern back into line.

Awake at night—tired next day?
P'raps your *Liver's* too wired, ("Let's play!")
If your ***Shen*** suffers doubt
Or your *Kidney's* bombed out,
You won't sleep, so have treatment—OK?

In addition to the organ/function diagnosis, Chinese medicine understands that each of the twelve major *meridians* has a time of peak activity every day. This may be taken into account in the treatment of insomnia, especially if someone routinely wakes suddenly at a certain time of night or can only sleep after, for instance, 3 am. Acupuncturists trained in the *Five Element* system, particularly, have a series of treatments for time-specific nocturnal waking.

And, finally, there is an 'extra' point, ***Anmian***, which translates as *Peaceful Sleep*. It's not on a regular *meridian* pathway, and it's often used to help in the treatment of insomnia. While we may choose to add this wonderful point during a treatment, we'll always make an overall assessment of a patient's diagnosis in order to help the person overcome sleeplessness, from a holistic viewpoint. If the cause is treated, the sleep problem is more likely to be helped long-term, not just temporarily.

You say ***Anmian*** helps me to sleep,
And will aid me to doze and go deep
Into dreamland (that's great:
It's been missing of late)
And will calm, head to toes—quite a feat!

It's important to note that Chinese medicine is very broad in the use of terms like *Heart*, *Kidney* and *Liver*. As I explained regarding the *Liver*, there is more to it than just the usual functions listed in Western medicine. Similarly, if your acupuncturist says, "I'm treating you for a ***Shen*** disturbance, which is related to your *Heart Spirit*", don't panic! It doesn't necessarily mean you have a physical heart problem (though, of course, some people do have heart problems), but it might mean that you are feeling emotionally ungrounded. And don't be alarmed by talk of the *Kidney* function: it doesn't mean you're heading for dialysis. There are all sorts of reasons for your practitioner to want to nourish your *Kidney* function, within the whole pattern of your treatment.

Backache

Does your backache go straight to your hip
Or your leg, with a nasty, sharp nip?
Is it better to walk,
Or would that make you baulk
And feel weak, or go arse over tip?

Backache is another problem that has many causes, and we make our diagnosis according to various factors, including the position and nature of the discomfort. For instance, a sharp pain that occurs in the hip would be treated differently from a dull ache in the same area, and an ache in the lumbar region would be treated differently again.

Other pointers towards different treatment strategies would be whether heat or cold makes a difference (maybe better or worse, in either case), whether movement improves or worsens the condition and whether the person is very tired… or short-tempered… or even whether they have cold knees.

Some lower backache is closely connected with the *Gall Bladder meridian*, some with the *Bladder meridian*, and some types are associated with the *Kidney meridian*.

When your knees feel so cold, and what's more,
Your lower back's achingly sore,
I'm warning you, Sidney,
Take care of your *Kidney*—
This story is old Chinese lore.

The kidney function affects the strength of the lower back, partly because it is responsible for the health of the body's battery pack (low battery = low power = low strength around the kidney area). Getting cold around this area depletes the *Kidney* energy. Consequently, we have predictable conversations with teenagers, which go something like this:

Doctor Pins: Hi, nice top.

Teenager: Thanks.

Doc Pins: Nice belly button piercing. I like the sparkly bit.

Teenager: Thanks.

Doc Pins: Do you often wear short tops like that, which expose your lower back?

Teenager: Yeah.

Doc Pins: Does your back get cold?

Teenager: Course not... anyway all my friends dress like this, too.

Doc Pins: Yep, and I think it looks great. My only concern is that your kidneys will get cold if you dress like that all year round... you might get a lot of colds, or perhaps cystitis or backache. You might even start to get some fat around there, as your body makes more fat in places it needs to protect.

Teenager: I get quite a lot of colds, but I promise you, that's not the reason. I don't feel the cold, even during a long night out.

Doc Pins: OK. I guess you're not too

bothered about getting short on battery power and a bit tired when you get older, either?

Teenager: No, I'm fine. I don't get tired.

Doc Pins: Well, I do have to advise you to keep warm around the middle when the weather's cold.

Teenager: Sure.

Doc Pins: So, now I've done my duty as an acupuncturist and given you my advice, and I guess that means you'll do your duty as a teenager, and ignore me...

Teenager: Yeah. Cool. (Grin.)

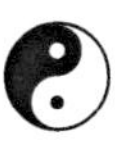

The Bee's Knees (and other joints)

My knees are so creaky, they seize,
And so swollen, on no account squeeze.
But please straighten each up
With three needles, one *cup*—
To help them become the bee's knees.

Joint pain can be really debilitating and in many cases it's something that acupuncture can help very effectively. Whether the pain is from a degenerative disease (like arthritis) or from an injury, we'll take a full medical history and ask you questions relating to the type of pain you experience. As well as asking how long you've had the problem, we'll want to know things like whether you have sharp pain or an ache, whether heat or cold makes it better or worse, whether the weather affects the pain, and so on.

Your answers to these questions help to ascertain the causes of your problems. Additionally, we'll take your pulses and look at your tongue, to improve the diagnosis and treatment strategy.

It's quite likely that we'll choose to use acupuncture points to help your overall health, and local points to bring more healing energy (***Qi***) directly to the places where you experience discomfort. For example, if you have knee pain, you might have some needles near to your ankles or wrists, as well as near to your knees.

You might also receive some other traditional Chinese treatment techniques, such as ***moxibustion*** and *cupping*, which are explained in the next two chapters.

Is it frozen or aching, your shoulder?
I ask, though I might still be bolder
And let treatment begin,
With a *cup* and a pin,
Or some ***moxa,*** to warmingly smoulder.

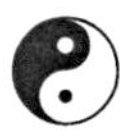

Moxibustion ~ Burning Herbs

Burning ***moxa*** goes right to the heart
Of the *Cold* in your body—that's smart.
Herbs, when shredded and dried,
Make you warm (but not fried)
And you won't end up cooked like a tart.

Moxibustion, or ***moxa***, has been used for centuries in China. ***Moxa*** is a shredded and dried herb of the *Artemisia* family. The herb itself has warming properties when used as an internal remedy. To increase the warming effect further, acupuncturists light it and let it smoulder close to patients, in several different, safe ways.

In acupuncture, a diagnosis that includes *Cold invasion* in the body means that we need to select acupuncture points that have a warming quality. The addition of ***moxa*** creates more warmth, faster. If you're a cold person, this feels lovely.

Moxibustion can be used in several different ways. One way is that it is made into small cones, and each cone, in turn, is placed over an acupuncture point. The top of the cone is then lit, to smoulder, and is removed as soon as the patient says, "Hot", which will be before the burning part gets to the skin. This is comfortably warming and safe. A similar method also uses cones, which are burned on a slice of ginger that buffers the heat from the skin.

Many practitioners use a method called *warm needle*, in which a small roll of ***moxa,*** wrapped tightly in paper, is placed securely on a needle and then burned. This is a very effective way of conducting the warmth directly to the acupuncture point.

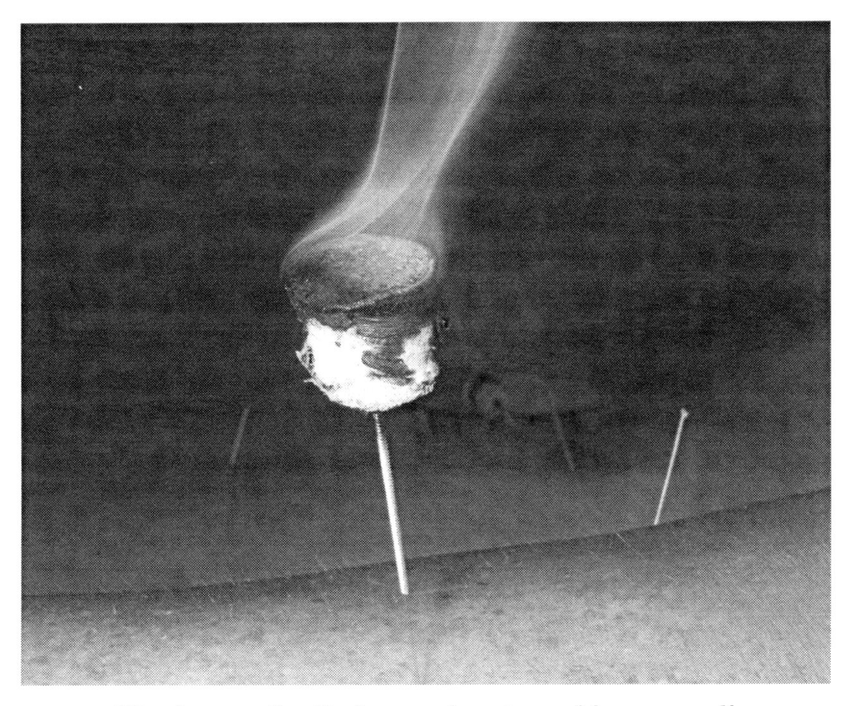

Here's a small roll of moxa burning safely on a needle

In China it's used far and wide,
And in various ways is applied:
On a needle or cone,
Burning all on its own
Or on salt, to get warmth deep inside.

There are two less usual ways of using ***moxa***.

If someone is very run down, we might use ***moxa*** on the point that is in the middle of the navel. This is a point that is forbidden for use with a needle or direct ***moxa***, so we fill the navel with salt, and burn the ***moxa*** cones on top of the salt, which insulates the delicate skin of this area.

And then there's the ***moxa box***... So much smoke billows out of these devices that, one time when I was in China, an English colleague, who works for the NHS, walked into the clinic and said, a little crossly, "I didn't think we were allowed to cook soup on our patients!" A wooden box that contains insulation and a raised grid is placed on the skin and a great pile of ***moxa*** is burned inside to give an extra amount of warmth to a cold or painful area, often on the lower back or the abdomen. This device is most frequently used with menstrual and fertility problems, and with severe backache.

A thing that quite frequently shocks
Is a bonfire of herbs, which unlocks
That sore pain in your back
(With no need for a rack).
Hot and smoky, a ***moxa*** box rocks!

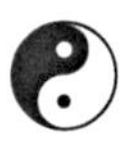

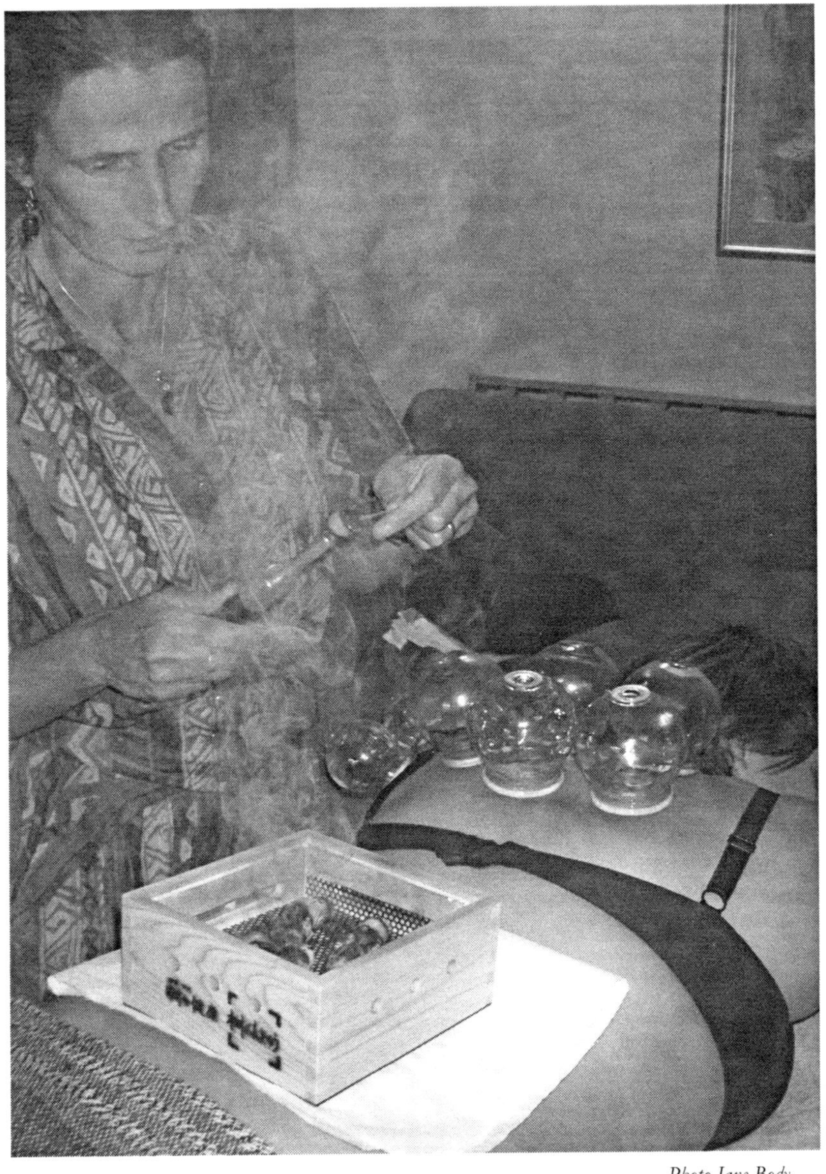

Photo Jane Body

Here the author is charging up a moxa box on a patient who already has cups on her back

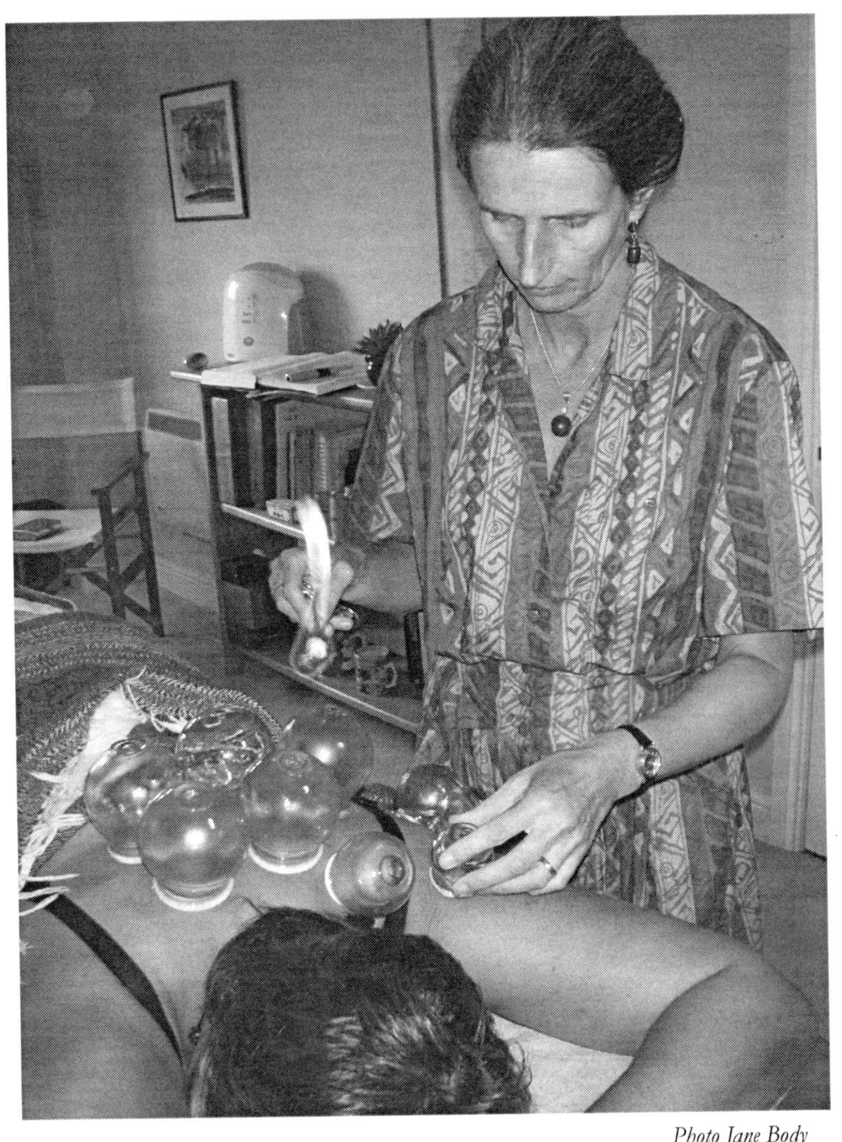

Photo Jane Body

Putting cups on a patient's shoulder

The Art of Cupping

If your shoulder pain's set to derange,
Or your backache needs serious change,
Then see Doctor Pins,
Whose *cupping* begins
With a flame in a jar—oh, how strange.

Yes, *cupping* is a technique that uses flame and a glass or bamboo cup to ease your aches and pains, move stagnation, and more.

The acupuncturist uses a lighted swab to create a vacuum in a *cupping jar*, which is then placed swiftly on the patient's sore muscle or joint. The flame on the swab is wafted into the *cup* to burn out some of the oxygen, and then it's removed again. So, when the *cup* is placed on the patient, no flame stays inside. However, the *cup* does remain soothingly warm.

A bubble of glass with a flame,
Makes a vacuum to stick… what a game!
It may seem like a circus,
But wait, please don't shirk us:
Not alarming, but calming… it's tame.

The vacuum has the effect of raising a small amount of flesh, which eases tension and stagnation, and so reduces pain. This is effectively like a massage in reverse, as a massage pushes the muscle in, whereas *cupping* slightly pulls it. Sometimes massage oil is used under a *cup*, so that it can be moved around to create a gentler treatment. This is often used if a patient is very weak or has been traumatised by, for instance, an accident.

If comfort's a thing that you lack
Accept *cupping* to ease your sore back,
And for lowered immunity
Have *cups* with impunity,
Once your therapist masters the knack.

Cupping is great on sore shoulders, backs and knees. If a person has enough flesh in the area, a tiny *cup* can even be used on a painful elbow. Sometimes a special technique is used, in which a little water is placed in the *cup* before it's applied, so it becomes a cooling treatment for someone with hot or inflamed joints. This can make the whole thing even more like a circus skill, as the practitioner has to remove the *cup* very quickly, with a flick of the wrist, and a lot of mop-up paper at the ready! This particular technique is not used so often…

We also use *cupping* to help support the body at times when the body's immunity is low, such as at the beginning of a common cold. Whatever you think about this, it certainly feels lovely to have warm cups placed on your upper back if you're coming down with a respiratory bug.

Some cups are bamboo; some are glass,
But if none is to hand, could you pass
Me a mug or a honey pot
To place on the funny spot?
This works, though it's lacking in class.

Normally, special round glass *cupping jars* are used, and in China, bamboo *cups* are frequently used. But if you don't have the right kit with you it's possible to achieve a good result with most cup-sized vessels, such as household mugs or jam jars. Consequently, many different 'looks' have been created in emergencies!

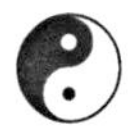

Five Types of Spirit

In the body, the spirit is ***Po***,
And ***Yi*** lets the intellect know
That the will is called ***Zhi***,
While the ***Hun*** serves to stir
The ***Shen*** into running the show.

In Chinese medicine, five of the functions/organs are seen as the homes of five different manifestations of spirit. Some of these are what we in the West might understand as spirit, and some are more akin to functions of the mind.

The spirit that relates to the *Heart* function/organ is the ***Shen***. This is the spirit of the consciousness of the mind and it also has the job of looking after all the other spirits. The ***Hun*** is the *Liver* spirit and is the spirit of hopes and dreams, and after death it lives on, so perhaps this is the one we might see as the heavenly spirit. The *Lung* spirit, the ***Po***, is, similarly, a subtle spirit, but it goes back to the earth at death. The ***Yi*** (pronounced *yee*) belongs to the *Spleen* and is to do with intellect, and the ***Zhi*** (pronounced *jehr*) lives with the *Kidneys* and is connected with willpower.

Shen ~ Heart

When your spirit desires to roam
And escape from your cranial dome,
Take good care of your ***Shen***,
'Cos it leaves the *Heart* when
There are lights on, but no-one's at home.

As in Western medicine, in Chinese medicine, the *Heart* is strongly associated with the *Blood*. It's said that having enough *Blood* enables us to have a stable mental and emotional state, and that the ***Shen*** or *Heart spirit* is responsible for maintaining this. Clear thinking, sharp memory and good sleep are all partially dependent on having stable ***Shen***. Chinese doctors look at a person's eyes to see into the soul, or assess the spirit. Dull, lifeless eyes (or sometimes eyes that sparkle **too** much) are seen as a sign of ***Shen*** disturbance.

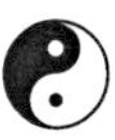

Hun ~ Liver

Creative, the ***Hun*** brings a shiver
Of plans full of hope: it's the giver
Of aims for a goal.
The ethereal soul
Is anchored by *Blood* in the *Liver*.

The ***Hun*** is translated from Chinese as the ethereal soul. It is seen as the mind-spirit, and is housed in the *Liver*. The ancient Chinese said that the ***Hun*** comes into our body three days after birth and deals with our capacity for planning and ideas.

To prevent these ideas from wandering off too fancifully, the ***Hun*** needs to be firmly rooted in the substance of the body, notably in the rich blood supply in the *Liver*. If the *Liver Blood* is deficient, the person can become dreamy in an uncentred way. This can lead to disturbed dreaming at night, as the ***Hun*** wanders too far from the body. An extreme example of this would be in a case of haemorrhaging, in which case Chinese medicine says that a person does not have enough *Liver Blood*, and consciousness temporarily leaves for dreamland: they are simply not able to stay in their body at this time, but their ethereal spirit or ***Hun*** is still sending images. So this partially explains the out-of-body experiences we sometimes hear about.

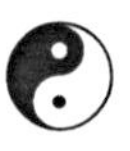

Po ~ Lung

The breath and the *Lungs* have in tow,
The corporeal soul, called the ***Po***.
Right from birth, it's around—
Then at death goes to ground,
Taking essence of life down below.

As well as the ***Hun***, which is the spirit that lives on after the death of the body, we have an earthly, bodily spirit that dies with us. This is associated with the *Lungs*, which house the breath of life, and affect our feelings. This piece of the soul, the ***Po*** (corporeal soul), is particularly affected by grief and sadness, and it has a strong connection with our essence, which, in Chinese medicine, is a tremendously important part of our vitality.

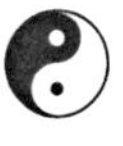

Yi ~ Spleen

If your everyday energy's slow,
And you study, but memory's low,
To keep intellect keen
You must tonify *Spleen*,
So your ***Yi*** can stay sharp—in the know.

Studying is a *Spleen* activity. If *Spleen* energy is low, the ***Yi*** *(Yee)*, the spirit housed in the *Spleen*, is also low, and the capacity to concentrate, remember and focus will also be tricky. Chinese students are made aware that too much study will injure the *Spleen* and they are encouraged to eat *Spleen-tonifying* food, such as naturally sweet root vegetables and liquorice root.

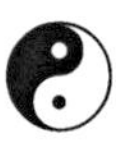

Zhi ~ Kidney

When life's challenges have you enthused,
You're determined—your will power's well used.
With your *Kidneys* so strong,
You'll be carried along
By your ***Zhi***—with no slacking excused!

The *Kidneys* house the 'spirit' of willpower or ***Zhi*** *(jehr)*. Strong *Kidney* energy is strong battery-power, so we have the will to move confidently towards our goals. If the *Kidneys* are exceptionally weak, we may not even muster the energy to have goals. Interestingly, this explains why we often don't have enthusiasm for anything after a bad illness, because the sickness has caused our body to have to delve deep into our battery-pack (*Kidney* ***Qi***) to try and find the energy to recover. This means that we don't have the spare capacity for the 'luxury' of being enthusiastic.

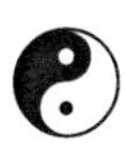

There are quite a few crossover points in the actions of the five spirits. Several have different connections to the memory, the sleep, the *Blood*, concentration and so on. A person who has problems in any of these areas may have issues with one or more of the relevant functions/organs. Part of the acupuncturist's skill is to decide which is the most vital in any one treatment.

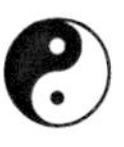

The Big Chill Out…

There was a young lady from Devon,
Who worked too hard, twenty-four seven.
When she wanted a chill-out,
Her bliss would soon spill-out—
Acupuncture—relaxing and heaven!

Yes! The really good news is that acupuncture can help you to chill out. This may be your main reason for having treatment, or it may be a rather nice 'side effect' of having treatment for a physical illness.

Maybe you just have too much to do in your life, or too much stress. Or perhaps you're facing a job interview or exams.

A young lady, called Jess, from the West,
Found exams caused her stress (at the best).
But this girl was no fool:
Acupuncture was cool,
And helped Jess face each test with more zest.

If you're nervous about something, or perhaps you have a phobia, get some treatment—don't wait any longer! If your lack of relaxation leads to a short fuse, you might end up being treated for ***Liver Qi Stagnation*** or ***Liver Yang Rising.*** Diagnostically, these are both syndromes of the Liver function, and if your energy is unbalanced in this way, a good acupuncture treatment, which addresses these problems, can leave you feeling surprisingly mellow.

Shock and trauma have an immediate and a long-lasting effect on your energy and well-being. Of course, one of the problems with shock is that, in order to try and normalise things as quickly as possible, your mind says, "No problem!" So it's quite usual to have a patient come in for some other issue and only then be treated to help resolve the shock in the system.

If you're dreading that aeroplane flight,
Or you're grumpy and itching to fight,
Or you're shocked to the core,
And can't take any more,
Chinese medicine can brighten your plight.

There are some really wonderful acupuncture points to treat shock and help with relaxation. ***Yin Tang***, which, translated from the Chinese, means *Hall of Impression*, is, as the name suggests, connected with our impressions, or emotional response to what life brings. So treating ***Yin Tang*** can significantly calm down your level of anxiety: it's one of the big chill-out points. Positioned in the middle of the forehead, just above the eyebrows, this is the point that is often shown on beautiful young models in photographs in newspaper articles or on brochures for health farms. The models always look very relaxed, which is quite correct!

Another point that is used frequently for treating shock is called ***Shen Men***, or *Spirit Gate*. It's a very fundamental point on the *Heart meridian*, and is gentle but powerful.

While these treatments for shock can be used on their own in emergency situations, we often use them in the context of complete acupuncture treatments, which are aimed at helping the whole person. This means that, while the immediate trauma is being addressed, the underlying problems are also being treated, so old patterns of illness and trauma are being reduced at the same time.

"Can you help me to chill and relax?
My composure is something that lacks."
"Let's treat ***Yin Tang*** to start,
And then ***Shen Men*** on *Heart*,
And do more than just paper the cracks."

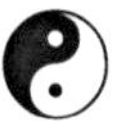

Fertility and Pregnancy

If pregnancy keeps slipping by
And conception has failed (don't know why),
An adjustment of ***Qi***
Might set your womb free
From the trouble that's making you sigh.

Chinese medicine has a good track record for helping women (and men) with fertility issues. Each person seeking help is individually diagnosed and treated, possibly for a deficiency of the *Kidney* function or an obstruction in the *Conception Vessel*. Or perhaps the abdomen is too cold to provide a good environment for conception to take place.

Diagnoses of *Cold* and *Damp* in the system are big issues in Chinese medicine, as the correct conditions are understood to be essential for efficient functioning of the body chemistry.

Because it is free of side effects, acupuncture is a very popular option for the various problems that can beset even the happiest, healthiest woman in pregnancy. Morning sickness, cramps, haemorrhoids, backache—even moodiness—can all be treated successfully.

When pregnancy's bumping along,
Acupuncture has points that are strong
For sickness and *Damp*,
And backache and cramp,
And emotions that somehow feel wrong.

Towards the end of a pregnancy, discovering that the baby is the wrong way up (in breech position) can lead to anxiety about the birth, or even to a caesarean section. A tiny acupuncture point called ***Zhi Yin*** *(Jehr Yin, Reaching Yin)* or *Bladder 67*, which is on the little toe, frequently solves this problem. It isn't needled. ***Moxa*** is burned over the point to warm it, and it can encourage the baby to move into the more usual 'launch position' of head-down.

When your baby's in breech, then let's add a
New option that's really no madder
Than Caesarean birth,
Using ***moxa*** that's worth
It on point 67 on *Bladder*.

If her baby is overdue and a woman is facing chemical or mechanical induction for the birth, she might opt for a less-invasive induction using acupuncture.

After the birth some women are unfortunate enough to suffer from post-natal depression. No one should ever underestimate how awful this is for a woman who is trying to be a good mother to a new baby. Chinese medicine has an approach, simultaneously pragmatic and sympathetic, as this dreadful condition is observed to have physical causes, which can be adjusted with knowledgeable treatment.

If your due date was ten days ago,
Or your labour is going too slow
(Or the post-partum blues
Come as terrible news)
Acupuncture's the best way to go.

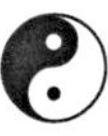

Ear Seeds ~ Nothing to Do with Gardening

~

That strange dot in my ear is a seed…
There are several to press when I need
To feel chilled or sustained,
Or when hunger has gained
Too much hold on me—is that agreed?

The human ear has an extraordinary number of acupuncture points on its surface.

Some practitioners use tiny acupuncture needles in the ears, but more often these points are used to support the patient between treatments. To do this we use minute seeds. Each one is stuck in place over an ear *acu* point with a very small square of plaster. Either real seeds from a Chinese plant called vaccaria, or tiny metal balls are used. The vaccaria seeds are naturally slightly irritating, so they stimulate the point, and the metal balls are often magnetic and have a similar effect. These can also be gold plated (though the 'bling' jewellery effect is lessened by the plaster over the gold seed!)

If your practitioner puts seeds in your ears to help support you between treatments, you will be asked to press them for a few moments several times a day, to increase the effect.

Ear seeds are often used to support the organs and relieve stress and to help with giving up smoking or with dieting.

Tiny balls in my ear help to bring
Gentle comfort and health—here's the thing:
All these small squares of plaster
Could help me heal faster—
Each fixing a seed... or some bling!

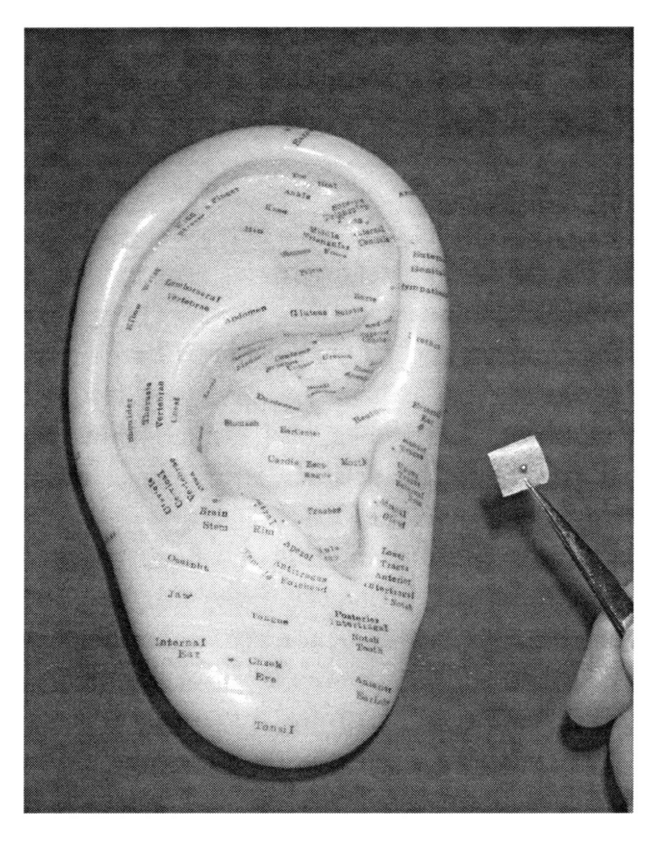

A plastic model for locating ear points, and a magnetic ear seed on a plaster

akupunkture kan b kool 4 kidz!

When treating those kids who have attitude,
Don't ever resort to a platitude—
But be there for real
As they grumble and squeal,
And accept that you'll not get much gratitude!

Yes, kids do come for treatment … and sometimes their parents would like them to and they refuse! There can be many reasons for children and young people to have acupuncture, such as exam nerves, asthma and allergies, frequent colds, tummy troubles, headaches, hormonal skin problems, menstrual pain, injuries, aches… and, yes… attitude and mood swings.

Kids are more likely than adults to have 'attitude' about coming for treatment. However, once they're comfortable with what probably started out as a very unknown experience, they can be surprisingly enthusiastic about acupuncture. They often find it 'well cool', and are frequently more sensitive than adults to what's going on in their energy.

Another very nice thing about kids and teenagers receiving treatment is that, because they usually have a shorter history of illness and trauma, there's a good chance that their initial recovery will be quicker than it is for adults.

Then you may be surprised and impressed
To be told that your treatment is best,
But please don't be depressed
If they're sassy (at best)...
Just remember that kids can be stressed.

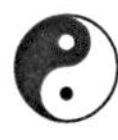

Acupuncture to Improve Your Looks… Too Good to Be True?

My friend, Nance, wants some pins to enhance
Her face, before Saturday's dance,
But the needling for Nancy
Will need to be fancy,
To advance her the chance of a glance.

Oh, poor Nancy: it doesn't sound as though there's much hope for her, does it? But while it's true that facial revitalisation (cosmetic) acupuncture won't turn an ordinary-looking person into a Hollywood look-alike, it can do a great deal to bring a healthy glow to a person's face and improve the skin quality, and some people find it even reduces wrinkles. So, actually, there's a good chance that Nancy will end up looking more attractive after all… though it won't necessarily all happen in one session, so let's not hold our breaths for this Saturday!

As we age (sadly, from about thirty-five onwards), the cells throughout our bodies gradually dehydrate. The effect this has on our looks is that our skin, hair and nails become drier and our eyes lose some of their shine. Tiny needles are used in facial revitalisation treatment, and the points selected help to bring ***Qi***, or life force, to the face, which helps cells to regain some of their moisture and energy.

While, mostly, we are afraid of words like 'plump', this is exactly what we want in our cells, as a plump cell is a happy and healthy cell. So by bringing more ***Qi*** to the cells of the facial skin, we encourage them to become more vibrant, which is what helps to increase radiance. This refers to the tiny cells within the skin; it does **not** mean the face will become fat!

Bringing ***Qi*** is the thing for the face:
It's reviving and laden with grace,
So leave botox behind—
Out of sight, out of mind—
Tiny needles help calm age's pace.

In addition to gently needling carefully selected points on the face, we treat the patient holistically, so we also select certain body points. This enhances the facial treatment and also means that you will gain some extra balance in your overall health while receiving a boost to your facial energy. This is important, as acupuncture is a system of medicine that affects the whole body-mind-spirit.

One final and interesting point about facial treatment is that our faces hold the visible memory of many of our past stresses and traumas. As acupuncture starts to work on the wrinkles and frown lines, the memory of old disturbances may start to shift out of the system, so it can actually help us to come to terms with past events in our lives, as cells let go of *body memory*.

I only came in for my face:
To smooth those old wrinkles and place
Such a bright healthy glow
That my beauty would show—
Now I'm feeling a new, deeper grace.

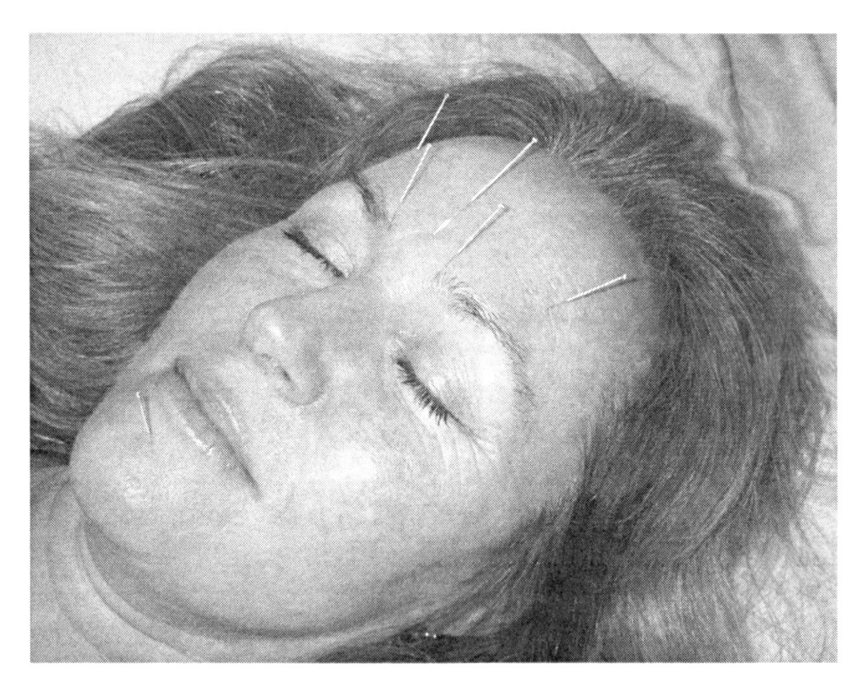

Facial Revitalisation Acupuncture

Interlude...

As I stand with this needle quite near
To your skin, you have nothing to fear,
And there's no need to scowl,
For I won't make you howl—
Am I making myself crystal clear?

Lots of us are real scaredy cats when it comes to teeny-weeny little acupuncture needles! But it's so far removed from the experience of something like an injection or a blood test, there's really no comparison. Yes, you should feel the needle hit the point, but you'll feel it as a unique electrical sensation, rather than what we would normally call pain.

So hang in there, and dare to try it. You'll find acupuncture extraordinary and helpful!

Anti-smoking and Weight Loss Treatments

To help the reduction of craving,
This treatment supports you by staving
Off needs and desires,
As it gently rewires
Your mind to rethink, without raving!

You may have heard about the use of acupuncture to help in reducing craving for cigarettes and aiding weight-loss. Because it helps to strengthen the health of the body-mind-spirit, regular 'everyday' acupuncture may encourage someone on the path to reducing weight or stopping smoking.

In addition to this holistic aspect, which is central to treatment, some practitioners will add special points to help shift the habit. Some of these points are in the ears, as well as the more usual locations.

Even if someone is having acupuncture to help them in the difficult task of changing a habit, they need to be committed to helping themselves as much as possible. For example, there is no point in having acupuncture (or any other treatment) to stop smoking if you have no plan to reduce the number of cigarettes smoked in a day.

Yes, it's true acupuncture can aid
Your big struggle with habits that played
A huge part in your day,
But there's **your** part to play,
As the fat melts or cigarettes fade.

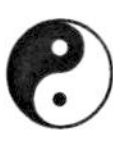

Smoking

Stop the fags? Really, guys, are you joking?
I'll say when I want to quit smoking!
So back off, you whacko—
I'll keep my tobacco—
Get lost with that needle… stop poking!

Exactly! There's no point in having any type of anti-smoking treatment until you want to stop. So the wise acupuncturist will always make sure that the hapless smoker in their consulting room is there of his or her own accord and not just because a partner or family member says they should be.

But, if and when you are ready to give up, your friendly local acupuncturist will do all they can to help. This may start with treatment to make you stronger in body, mind and spirit, so that your health and willpower are as resourced as possible. Then, while you are chilling out with needles in points for 'you', your practitioner may add tiny needles in ear acupuncture points and/or use ear seeds, which are weeny seeds or metallic balls under very small squares of sticking plaster. These ear seeds will stay in for up to a week, so that you can keep the treatment going by pressing them.

Your acupuncturist may even put the most miniscule semi-permanent needles into your ears, also under plaster, and also for you to press between treatments.

If you want to be rid of the habit,
When offered some treatment, go grab it.
Acupuncturists heed
Your great fight with the weed—
Simply offer your ear and we'll stab it!

...gently!

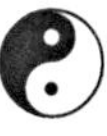

Weight Loss

You complain, "It's so very unfair!
All my skinny friends easily dare
To eat hugely, like horses,
And nobody forces
Their fare to be barely a pear."

It really **is** unfair. Some people have the cheek just to be thin, while others struggle with weight all the time. One of the great benefits of acupuncture is that it addresses metabolism as well as the energy level, so if someone is overweight because of a sluggish metabolism or under-active thyroid, it can aid improvement.

There is also the issue that many people have the *Pathogenic Factor, Damp,* in their bodies, which means they routinely hold extra fluid. Clearing *Damp* is a slow process, but one that acupuncture is equipped to tackle. This is described in the chapter on *Pathogenic Factors.*

If you find it hard to stop yourself eating too much, or even binging, acupuncture can help you to retrain your habits, because it balances your body-mind relationship. It is also quite likely that we'll put magnetic or natural seeds in your ears, as with the anti-smoking treatment, but we'll use some different points, notably adding ones to affect the stomach and appetite.

But, be warned, while treatment may help with weight, a few acupuncture needles won't cause weight to fall away instantly or without co-operation from you.

Are you feeling too heavy? Well, damn!
If you ask me to help you, I am
Quite prepared to assist
Your desire to desist
That habit to gobble and cram!

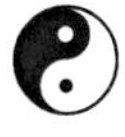

Drug Detox

Quitting drugs? Well you know it's no breeze,
So, when queasy or shaking, do please
Support de-tox with *NADA*,
Before it gets harder,
To get some calm moments of ease.

In 1972 a doctor in Hong Kong discovered that putting needles in five particular acupuncture points in the ears helped people to get over the symptoms of drug withdrawal more quickly. It also helps to relax people who are undergoing a process that can be nerve-wracking.

A specific set of ear points is used, and this is called the *NADA* protocol (*National Acupuncture Detoxification Association*) and, because the client does not necessarily have body acupuncture at the same time, sometimes this procedure is carried out by specially trained drug workers, who do not have to be acupuncturists. Even so, some drug projects employ fully trained acupuncturists to administer this protocol.

The five points used are ***Shen Men*** (*Spirit Gate*), which is a wonderful chill-out point, a second point to target the autonomic nervous system and three points for ***yin*** organs (the *Kidneys*, *Liver* and *Lungs*), because these organs are especially involved in de-toxifying the system.

To help with your de-tox, begin
With some ear needles, gently eased in,
To encourage and calm
Your hurt soul, like a balm:
Treat the nerves, *Spirit Gate* and the ***Yin***.

As with all treatments and support for recovering addicts, it is important to be aware that the acupuncture de-tox protocol is not going to 'make' the person stop their habit as though by magic. It is always essential that the addict should wish to stop. However, once they are going through the uncomfortable withdrawal process, the *NADA* protocol (possibly combined with more systemic acupuncture and other help, such as drug or alcohol counselling) can be deeply supportive as well as hastening the process of removing toxins from the body.

Drug de-tox protocol, using ear needles

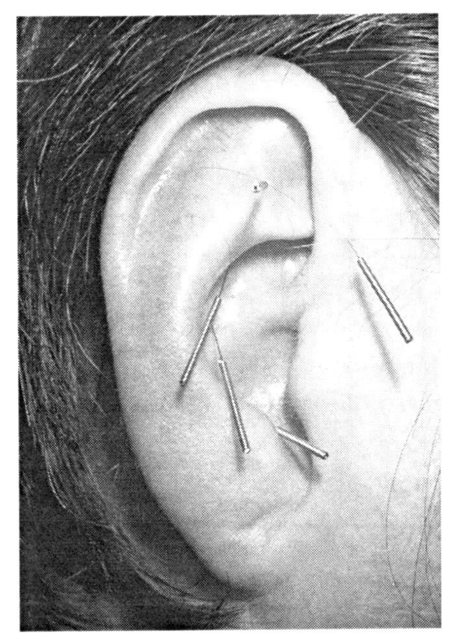

The Tyrolean Iceman

Deep in ice, an old body was found,
Well preserved, with tattoos, now renowned:
Most especially some points
That would help his sore joints
In three thousand BC… how profound!

We know little about this old iceman—
A slow coach, or done-in-a-trice-man?
Was he Stefan or Cyril,
This man from the Tyrol—
A warlord or simply a nice man?

Preserved for long years in a glacier,
The iceman's tattoos were far classier
Than 'Cyril loves Rose',
From his head to his toes…
He had dots and designs so much sassier!

Join the dots, there are points, we can number,
To help his pain, gastric and lumbar.
Tattoos on the skin
Of the back and the shin—
Show his treatment before that long slumber.

A mummified body, dating from before 3,000 BC, was found preserved in a glacier near the Austrian-Italian border. It has tattoos on it, which accurately identify acupuncture points, well known (and named and numbered) in modern times. Nowadays those very same points might be used to treat the sorts of degenerative lower back and bowel problems evident in the body of that famous iceman.

How cool is that?

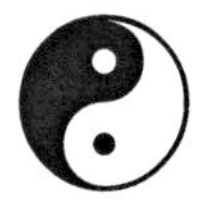

Resources

Further Reading

The Acupuncture Handbook by Angela Hicks: *Piatkus 2005*

How to find a qualified acupuncturist in your country

This list is not exhaustive, so please check the Internet for further contacts.

United Kingdom
British Acupuncture Council
Tel: 020 8735 0400
www.acupuncture.org.uk

Ireland
Acupuncture Foundation Professional Association
Tel: 01 412 4917
www.acupro.ie

Acupuncture Council of Ireland
Tel: National Locall Helpline: 1850 300 600
Dedicated phone line: 01 2393267
www.tcmci.ie

Canada
www.medicinechinese.com

Europe (all of Europe)
Pan European Federation of TCM Societies
Tel: +31 (0)20 689 2468
www.pefots.com

There are also country-specific professional associations throughout Europe.

Australia
Australian Acupuncture and Chinese Medicine Association
Tel: +61 (0)7 3324 2599
www.acupuncture.org.au

New Zealand
New Zealand Register of Acupuncturists
Tel: +64 (0)4 387 7672
0800ACUPUNCTURE [0800 228 786]
www.acupuncture.org.nz

USA
American Association of Acupuncture and Oriental Medicine
Tel: 916-443-4770
866-455-7999 Toll-Free
www.aaaomonline.org

South Africa
National Acupuncture and Chinese Medicine Association of South Africa (NACMASA)
Tel: (021) 697-0611/3 or (021) 696-9484
www.nacmasa.co.za

Gentle reader, please tell me we're winning –
Think back to that slender beginning:
Has all of my wheedling
Convinced you that needling
Can help you with life's underpinning?

&